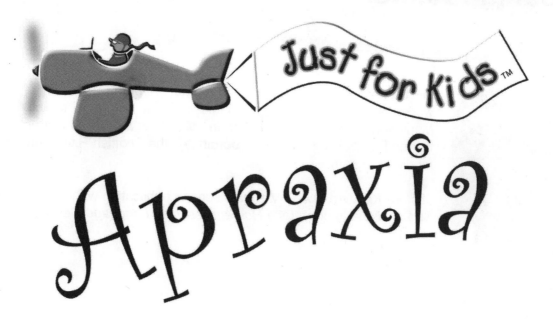

Apraxia

Just for Kids™

Martha Drake

Skill Area:	Apraxia
Ages:	4 thru 8
Grades:	PreK thru 3

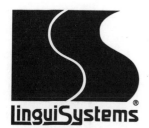

LinguiSystems

LinguiSystems, Inc.
3100 4th Avenue
East Moline, IL 61244-9700
1-800 PRO IDEA
1-800-776-4332

FAX: 1-800-577-4555
E-mail: service@linguisystems.com
Web: www.linguisystems.com
TDD: 1-800-933-8331
(for those with hearing impairments)

Printed in the U.S.A.
ISBN 0-7606-0353-7

About the Author

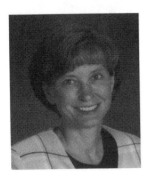

Martha Drake, M.A., CCC-SLP, is a graduate of the University of Iowa. She works as a speech-language pathologist in the outpatient clinic at Parkview Medical Center in Pueblo, Colorado. Martha is a certified instructor of the Hanen Parent Program. She coordinates the Scottish Rite Foundation funding program.

Just for Kids: Apraxia is Martha's second publication with LinguiSystems. She is also author of *Take Home: Preschool Language Development*.

Dedication

This manual is dedicated to the Scottish Rite Foundation of Colorado. Through their generosity, thousands of children have received the gift of effective communication.

Illustrations by Margaret Warner

Cover Design by Mike Paustian

Page Layout by Christine Buysse

Table of Contents

Introduction

Just for Kids: Apraxia is a practical and effective tool for working with children with developmental apraxia of speech in both individual and group therapy. The approach is based on solid therapeutic principles. The session sequence includes:

- a gross motor warm-up activity
- oral-motor exercises
- gestural cues
- drill in systematically more complex phonetic and linguistic contexts
- functional expressions
- family or aide practice activities

The advantage of *Just for Kids: Apraxia* is in its efficiency — it makes it easy for you to plan and manage the activities in the therapy session. The program can also be used effectively by an aide with your direction and supervision.

Group therapy is a reality. High caseloads, dwindling reimbursement, and demands on productivity have influenced how therapy is structured in most settings, whether it be a school, hospital, or a private clinic. Group therapy has therapeutic advantages also — children are challenged and reinforced by their peers, therapy occurs in a more naturalistic environment, and an informal support system is established. In group therapy, however, it is very difficult to effectively manage complicated task hierarchies, boundless therapy materials, and detailed response forms. Your attention must be focused on group dynamics.

Just for Kids: Apraxia uses the alphabet to organize the session. The alphabet thematically ties together the activities in the session sequence. Phonemes are drilled using flash cards presented in ABC order. (The phonemes /sh/, /ch/, and /th/ have been added to the end of the alphabet. The /zh/ phoneme is not included in the program because of its low frequency of occurrence.) Responses are scored on an alphabet response form. The alphabet is also a very practical tool for children, parents, and aides. They are familiar with it and understand its sequence and organization. Many children with apraxia of speech have difficulty learning to read and spell. An added advantage of using the alphabet in apraxia therapy is its positive impact on phonological awareness, reading, and writing skill development. In addition, alphabet-related materials are readily available for use in therapy and for home carryover activities.

How to Use the Program

The program is designed to be used with children ages 4 through 8. Begin by evaluating the children either informally or with a formal assessment tool prior to enrollment. An informal pre/posttest is included on pages 134 – 136 of the manual. Characteristics that distinguish children with developmental apraxia of speech from other speech disorders include:

- delayed in gross and fine motor coordination
- groping for sound placement
- able to produce sounds in isolation and short words, but longer utterances are unintelligible
- difficulty imitating oral movements
- slow, deliberate speech

- altered rhythm and intonation
- short utterances
- speaks mostly in vowels, bilabials, and stops
- inconsistent error patterns (not the typical /s/, /r/, /l/, and /k/ errors)
- poor response to traditional articulation therapy and phonological processes approach

The children should have prior knowledge of the alphabet, although they need not be proficient with it. If you are running a group, limit the size to three to five children. The suggested duration for sessions is 45 minutes to one hour. Distribute the Introductory Family Letter, page 12, at an orientation meeting prior to starting therapy. At that time, discuss the Home Practice Log and Home Practice Notes that will accompany family letters at the beginning of each phase and the importance of daily home practice. Children with developmental apraxia of speech need regular, intense drill in order to change their motor plans. Unfortunately, most of us do not have the luxury of working with these children on a daily basis. We need to enlist the help of family or classroom aides if available.

Start the session with a gross motor warm-up activity. You may want to begin in a gym area or perform the gross motor activity on the way to therapy (e.g., climbing stairs, marching, skipping, etc.). Conduct the session in an area free from visual and auditory distractions. The children should sit at a table in chairs that allow for good posture with their feet flat on the floor. For variation, have the children sit on a large therapy ball for all or part of the session. The proprioceptive feedback they receive from balancing themselves on a ball can improve their verbal response. Overall stability is important for good speech production.

Description of the Program

Developmental apraxia of speech is a motor speech disorder in which children have difficulty planning, executing, and sequencing the oral movements required for intelligible speech. As the phonetic and linguistic load of the message increases, speech intelligibility decreases. *Just for Kids: Apraxia* provides strategies and materials for working with children with apraxia in five phases:

- Phase One: Sounds in Isolation
- Phase Two: C-V-C Words
- Phase Three: Multisyllabic Words
- Phase Four: Sentences
- Phase Five: Expressions

Each phase of the program includes:

- rationale
- strategies
- criterion for moving to the next phase
- session sequence
- family letter and home practice materials
- supplemental target list
- reproducible ABC Flash Cards
- phase completion certificate

Introduction, continued

The book also includes:

- mouth posture pictures
- alphabet signs
- gross motor movement activities
- suggested reinforcement materials
- introductory family letter
- long- and short-term goals
- group and individual response forms
- progress report form
- program completion report form
- references

Rationale

A rationale is provided at the beginning of each phase. The purpose of the phase, the way it relates to other phases, typical error patterns, and performance expectations are addressed in this section.

Strategies

Specific strategies are provided for each phase to facilitate successful responses from the children. Although the strategies are listed by phases, they are meant to be cumulative in nature (i.e., strategies helpful in Phase One will also be appropriate to use in Phase Five).

Criterion for Moving to the Next Phase

It is recommended that all children achieve a 75-80% proficiency level before moving to the next phase of the program. Response accuracy is judged by the production of the whole utterance, not individual phonemes. In later phases of the program, linguistic and prosodic features are considered as well as articulation.

Instructional Tools

Alphabet Signs: Pictures of the manual sign language alphabet are provided on pages 13 – 17 to send home with the Introductory Family Letter and to use when learning the signs in the Alphabet Chant.

Alphabet Mouth Postures: Mouth posture pictures of the sounds of the alphabet are included on pages 139 – 147. Airflow, voicing, lip and tongue placement, and nasality are shown on the pictures. Use the alphabet mouth posture pictures for additional visual support when performing the Alphabet Chant and for difficult sound productions throughout the session.

Oral-Motor Mouth Postures: Each phase has mouth posture pictures to go with the oral-motor exercises. The pictures may help children with oral apraxia form more precise lip and tongue movements.

ABC Flash Cards: Each phase has a set of reproducible ABC Flash Cards. Use the flash cards in the drill portion of the session and send them home with the family letters for home practice. To avoid confusion for both you and the family, you may want to copy the flash cards on different colored paper. A laminated set is best for therapy. In addition to the target utterance, the flash cards also use the target in a more challenging context. Use the challenging context once the target is easily produced. The challenging contexts for each phase are as follows:

> *Phase One*: A word is provided that contains a syllable that sounds like the letter name.
> Target: **D**
> Challenging Context: dan**de**lion

> *Phase Two*: The C-V-C word is used in a short phrase or sentence.
> Target: **hot**
> Challenging Context: The soup is hot.

> *Phase Three*: The multisyllabic word is used in a carrier phrase.
> Target: **kitty cat**
> Challenging Context: I want a kitty cat.

> *Phase Four*: The sentence is followed by a question requiring the children to retain the linguistic and phonemic features of the utterance.
> Target: **He ran a race.**
> Challenging Context: What did he do?

> *Phase Five*: The expression is followed by a role-play situation requiring the children to retain the linguistic, phonemic, and prosodic features of the utterance for a longer period of time.
> Target: **Fe, fi, fo, fum!**
> Challenging Context: You are the giant in *Jack and the Beanstalk*. You smell the boy.
> What do you say?

Supplemental Target List: A supplemental list is provided with each phase. Use it as alternative stimuli to the targets on the flash cards or as additional practice items.

Family Letter and Home Practice Materials: Six family letters are provided in the manual. The Introductory Family Letter, page 12, describes the overall program and should be presented at an initial family overview meeting. Attach the Alphabet Signs, pages 13 – 17, to the Introductory Family Letter. Subsequent letters introduce each phase, providing a brief description of the phase and home practice suggestions. They should be distributed following the first session of each phase along with a copy of the ABC Flash Cards, Home Practice Log, and Home Practice Notes.

Phase Completion Certificate: A Phase Completion Certificate is included at the end of each phase. The certificate is intended as a reward for the children and to signal to parents/caregivers the start of a new phase in the program.

Clinical Tools

Pre/posttest: The informal assessment on pages 134 – 136 is provided to measure progress and response to treatment. It uses a simple +/– scoring system and assesses skills addressed in the program.

Response Forms: An Apraxia Group Response Form, page 151, and an Apraxia Individual Response Form, page 153, are included in the manual. An alphabet grid is used to record the accuracy of responses in all phases of the program. The forms have a +/– scoring system and a percent correct table. Completed forms are provided as samples following each response form.

Goals: Long- and short-term goals, page 150, are provided to assist you in writing treatment plans and individual educational plans.

Progress Report Form: Use the Progress Report Form, page 155, at any time in the program to share information with parents/caregivers, teachers, physicians, etc.

Program Completion Report Form: At the end of the program, use the Program Completion Report Form, page 156, to document and communicate response to therapy.

Therapy

Materials

The materials for each phase of the program are listed at the beginning of the unit.

Session Sequence

Gross Motor Warm-Up: The session begins with a gross motor warm-up activity to improve the children's overall coordination and to prepare them for success in oral-motor tasks. The children sing the ABC song in unison as they perform the gross motor activity. Combining speech with a gross motor movement may be very difficult for some children at first, but performance will improve over time. Sing the song slowly and with exaggerated articulation so the children can keep up with you. Repeat the song and movement activity several times. Encourage the children to watch your mouth for visual cues during all parts of the session.

Oral-Motor Exercises: Oral-motor exercises not only increase the strength and coordination of the speech musculature, but also give the children a greater awareness of where their articulators are in their mouths. The exercises will improve their ability to follow placement instructions for sounds. Three lip exercises and three tongue exercises are listed for each phase. The exercises have accompanying pictures. Model each exercise and ask the children to compare their movements with yours and with the pictures. Repeat each exercise as a group five times. It is difficult to count and model the exercise at the same time so use your fingers to indicate the number of repetitions.

Alphabet Chant: The manual sign language alphabet is used as a gestural cueing system throughout the program. The children learn the sign language alphabet in a chant, pages 137 – 138, which requires them to form the sign, say the letter name, and produce the associated sound(s). The goal is for the children to eventually use the alphabet signs as a self cue for difficult sounds in words. Lead the alphabet review by forming the manual letter sign as you say the sentence. Encourage the children to chime in. Some children may need hand-over-hand assistance to form the alphabet signs. Then show a graphic representation of the letter. This can be done by placing a magnetic letter on a board, writing the letter on a chalkboard, pointing to the letter on an alphabet chart, placing a letter puzzle piece in an alphabet puzzle, etc. You will find many alphabet materials commercially available or in the classroom to use in this activity. Develop a cadence to your alphabet review to enhance the children's responses. Pictures of the mouth postures for the sounds associated with the alphabet letters are provided on pages 139 – 147. Use these to teach and reinforce sound production. After the children have learned the manual signs and sound-letter associations, the alphabet review may be meshed with the drill portion of the session.

Drill: Drill is the most important part of the session. Children with developmental apraxia of speech need intensive and successful drill to change their motor plans. In each session, plan adequate time for drill and aim for a large number of responses. The most effective way to achieve this is through unison practice and a fast pace. Show the children the ABC Flash Card and then ask them to repeat the target with you as a group five times. Use your fingers to indicate the number of repetitions. Give manual letter cues and placement instructions when introducing the target. Fade in and out of the drill as needed. Following the unison practice, ask each child to produce the target individually. Try to drill all the ABC Flash Cards in each session. If a particular letter/sound is difficult, provide additional instruction and practice, then go on. Your goal is to practice the whole set of flash cards rather than dwelling on individual error sounds. You do not always need to start drill with the letter A. You may want to start from the back of the alphabet and move forward, or shuffle the flash cards for a random order. Another strategy is to start where you left off during the previous session so all targets have equal practice time. Record the accuracy of responses using +/– on the Apraxia Group/Individual Response Forms, pages 151 – 154. Remember that apraxia is a disorder of movement transitions. Move to a more complex phonetic or linguistic context whenever the child has successfully produced the target.

Most children will do what is expected of them. Do not present drill as something boring, but as an expectation. If you can avoid using a reinforcer in therapy, you will increase the number of responses possible during the session. Some children, especially younger children, need a tangible reinforcer to stay on task. Keep the reinforcer quick, uncomplicated, and related to the alphabet. Many alphabet related reinforcement materials are available commercially or may be borrowed from the classroom teacher. See page 149 for suggestions. Whenever possible, save the reinforcer for the end of the session. For example, place an ABC floor puzzle piece in a box after drilling each target and have the children assemble the puzzle as a group at the end of the session. Another way to reduce time spent on the reinforcement activity is to give the reinforcer after drilling three or four flash cards rather than after each flash card.

Words of Increasing Length: In this exercise, the children learn fun, dynamic expressions they can take back to the classroom or use at home. Ask the children to repeat the syllable groups until the entire utterance is produced. Hand gestures for "your turn/my turn" can help establish the echoing routine. After practicing the expression a few times, call on individual children to produce the utterance in a functional context. Suggested role plays are provided.

Song: Three popular children's songs are provided. Select one of these songs to wrap-up your session in a fun, functional way. Slow the rate so the children can attend to their speech production.

Closure: Invite parents/caregivers into the session to discuss progress towards goals, production cues, effective drill strategies, etc. Distribute the ABC Flash Cards, Family Letter, Home Practice Log, and Home Practice Notes at the beginning of each phase for daily practice at home. Suggest that the family members sing the song selected in therapy and read the books listed in the family letter with the child to facilitate carryover. The books are good children's literature that have a repetitive, sing-song quality to them. Family members should read the books slowly with exaggerated expression, pausing so the child can complete phrases and join in on refrains. The books are readily available at book-stores, libraries, and may even be in the classroom. Present the Phase Completion Certificate at the end of each phase.

Completion of the Program

The goal of *Just for Kids: Apraxia* is to develop intelligible, functional speech in children with developmental apraxia of speech. Their speech may not be error-free upon completion of the five phases. The following options are available and should be based on posttest results and clinical judgment:

- Schedule individual therapy to focus on specific needs.
- Cycle through some or all of the phases in the program a second time.
- Move to a traditional therapy or phonological processes approach.
- Continue to increase phonetic and linguistic complexity of targets (similar to the later stages in fluency therapy).

Adaptations for Special Needs Populations

Children with special needs such as Down syndrome, cerebral palsy, head injury, hearing impairment, cleft palate, etc., may have an apraxic component to their speech impairment. *Just For Kids: Apraxia* can be used very effectively with these children. More emphasis may need to be placed on oral-motor exercises due to the presence of a dysarthria. Do not delete the gross motor warm-up with physically impaired children; they need the physical and sensory input even more than other children for success on verbal tasks. Consult a physical or occupational therapist for special instructions on handling a child with physical limitations.

Individual therapy may be more effective than group therapy with children with special needs. Expect a longer and more intensive course of therapy to complete the program.

Conclusion

Working with children with apraxia of speech can be a challenging and often frustrating process. At times you wonder if the children will ever become effective verbal communicators. Hang in there! A thorough, systematic approach will pay off in the long run with most children. The joy of helping an unintelligible child speak clearly is well worth the effort!

Martha

Dear Family,

_____ will participate in apraxia therapy on
(child's name)

_____ from _____ to _____ .
(day/s)   (time)   (time)

Children with apraxia have difficulty planning and sequencing the movements needed for intelligible speech. Their speech typically breaks down as words and sentences become longer.

The approach I am using is based on the alphabet. The first step will be to say the letters of the alphabet clearly. The next step is to practice one-syllable words, then words with two to four syllables, then short sentences, and finally common expressions. The goal is to have your child speaking clearly in conversation by the end of the therapy program. The manual sign language alphabet will be used to cue difficult sounds. Please practice the attached alphabet signs.

At the beginning of each step of the program, I will send home a Family Letter, a Home Practice Log, Home Practice Notes, and a set of ABC Flash Cards. Please practice these flash cards every day with your child. Your child needs consistent practice to change any speech patterns. Briefly provide additional practice for any sounds that are difficult and then go on to the next card. Don't dwell on difficult sounds. Record the accuracy of your child's response as correct (+) or incorrect (−) on the Home Practice Log. Total the number of correct responses at the bottom of the column.

I will also provide book and song suggestions that reinforce each step of the program. The books are good children's literature and should be available at the library. Encourage your child to read the book along with you, joining in on the refrain or rhyming word. By slowing your rate and reading with exaggerated expression, you will help your child learn the necessary movements for speech. The songs are common children's songs. Ask me for the words if you need them. Sing the songs slowly so your child can join in.

Please call me if you have any questions or would like to schedule a time to observe therapy. I am looking forward to working with your child.

Sincerely,

_____
Speech-Language Pathologist

_____
Phone

Alphabet Signs

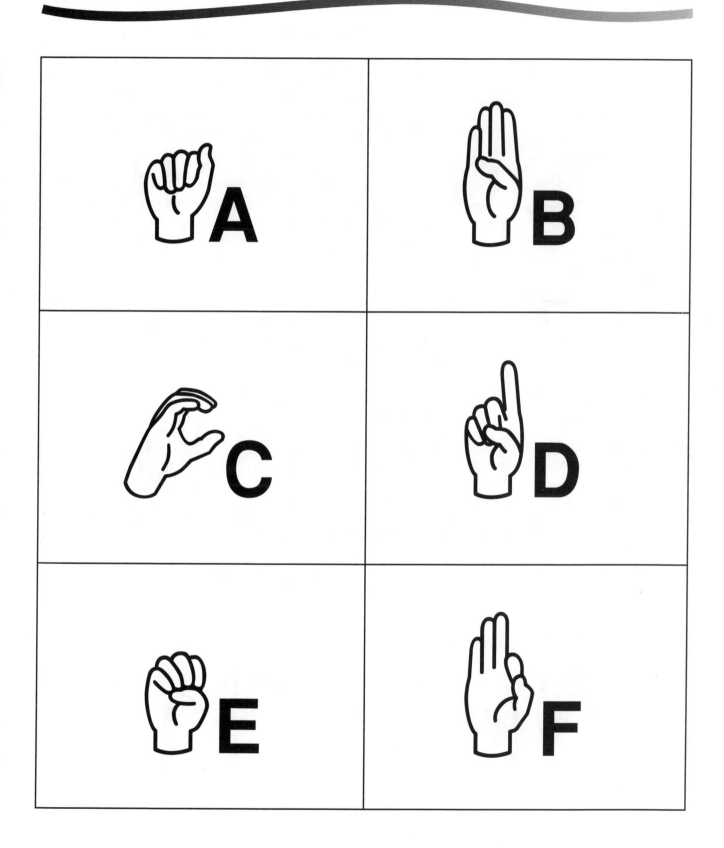

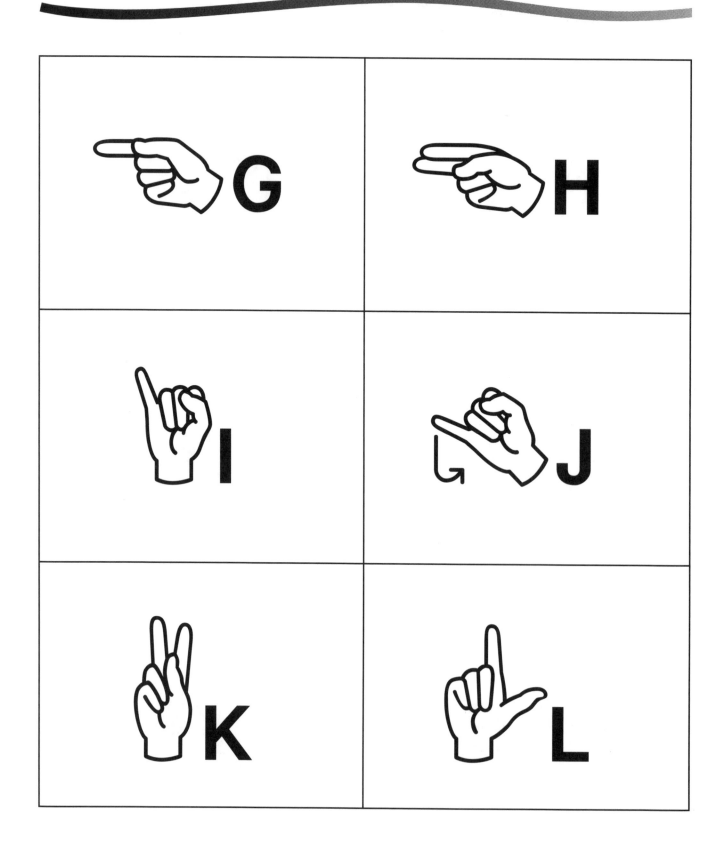

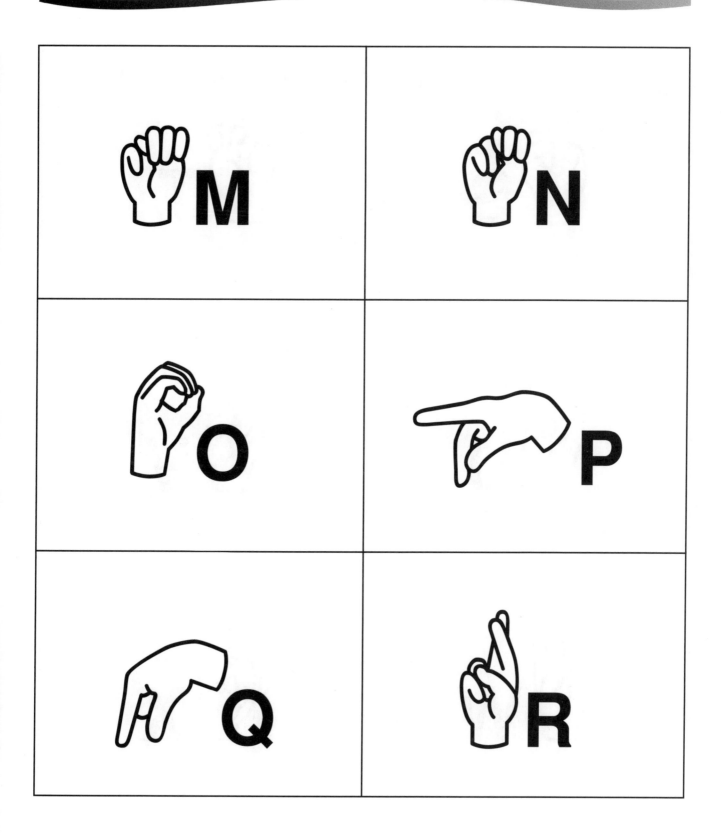

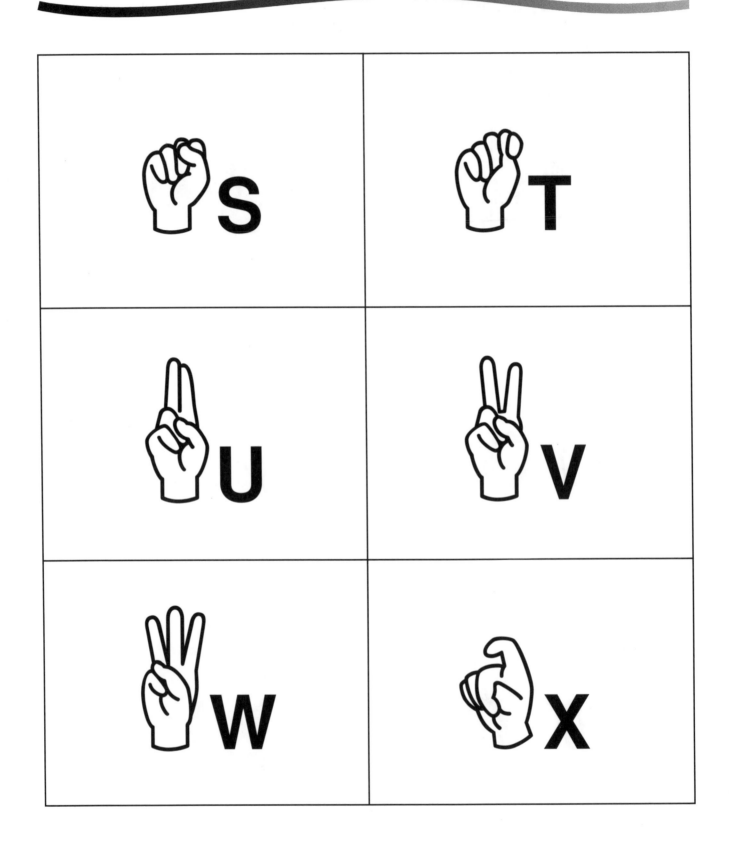

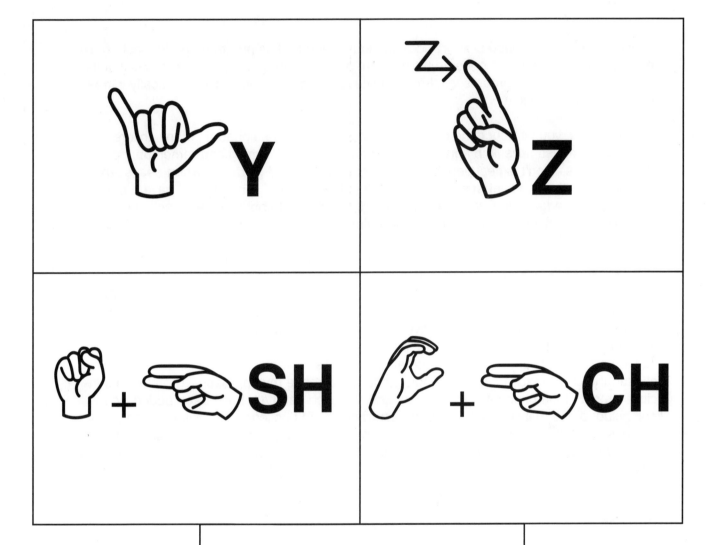

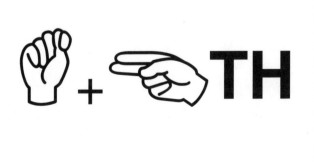

Sounds in Isolation
Phase One

Rationale

Sounds in Isolation: Phase One provides the foundation for this program. As in most apraxia therapy approaches, it is a bottom-up treatment plan. The program begins with small units (i.e., letter names) and progresses through levels in which the stimuli systematically increase in length and complexity.

In Phase One, you introduce the children to the sign language alphabet. Many children with verbal apraxia also have limb apraxia and will have difficulty forming and remembering the alphabet signs. Don't expect perfection. Use hand-over-hand guidance when necessary. Persistence with the alphabet signs will pay off in the long run. Children will have a more concrete knowledge of individual letters and will use the alphabet signs as a self-cue. You will have an effective nonverbal means for cueing sounds.

The children are required to pronounce letter names correctly in Phase One of the program. This is very different from most apraxia programs which focus on sounds, not letters. The sounds are traditionally organized by order of acquisition, place of articulation, manner of articulation, voiced-voiceless cognates, frequency of occurrence, or some other clinical dimension. From the child's perspective, however, sounds are not as meaningful as letters and our organizational schemes seem random. Teachers and parents expect children to say the alphabet clearly. Children need alphabet skills for reading and writing. So I have chosen the child/ teacher/parent-friendly alphabet to shape my approach. The alphabet includes most of the phonemes in our language (/sh/, /ch/, and /th/ have been added; /zh/ is not included due to its low frequency of occurrence.). To challenge the children when they can easily say the letter name, ask them to repeat the word pictured on the flash card. The pictured word has a sylla-ble in it that sounds like the letter name (e.g., the word *bumblebee* has the letter name B in *bee)*.

Strategies

Children with apraxia do not learn well through the auditory channel alone. A multisensory approach to learning is required. They need to:

- see the sound
- feel the sound
- hear the sound
- understand the sound

The strategies described on pages 19 – 21 will be helpful in Phase One.

See the Sound

- Do not present a verbal stimulus until everyone is watching your mouth.

- Frequently redirect children to watch your mouth. A pause followed by pointing to your mouth is often more effective than using words.

- "Get in the child's face" if he resists looking at your mouth. Try gently holding his head in your hands if he has difficulty focusing on facial cues.

- Encourage children to match their mouth posture either with yours or with another child's. (Using another child as a group model is very motivating. Everyone wants to be the expert!)

- Show pictures of the Alphabet Mouth Postures on pages 139 – 147. The light bulb indicates that the voice is "on." Nasality is indicated by a shaded dot on the nasal bridge. Airflow is represented by lines for continuants and a cloudburst for stops. Some sounds have more than one mouth posture, like Q, X, and some vowels. To make these sounds, the mouth moves from one posture to the other.

- Describe how a sound looks (e.g., "Your tongue is up," "Your lips are closed," "Your mouth is open," etc.).

- Use a mirror. Give each child a small hand-held mirror to use when they need additional visual feedback.

Feel the Sound

- Explore how the sound feels. Describe the feel of the sound using dynamic action words such as *squeezing*, *buzzing*, *tapping*, etc.

- Discuss the degree of tension in the jaw, lip, and tongue muscles (e.g., "Your lips are loose," "Squeeze your tongue," "Tighten your jaw," etc.).

- Present stimuli slowly and with exaggerated movements. Children with apraxia need extra time to process, plan, and feel speech movements.

Hear the Sound

- Bombard the children with auditory models.

- Use nonverbal cues (e.g., alphabet signs, pages 13 – 17; mouth posture pictures, pages 139 – 147) and reinforcement (e.g., okay sign, thumbs-up, head nod). These cues are quicker and do not overload the children's auditory systems.

- Control interfering background noise.

Understand the Sound

- Use imagery and pretend play to give the sound meaning. Young children often do not have the concept of a sound or a letter. By providing a familiar sound and attaching it to a letter, they begin to develop sound-symbol associations. Use the following imagery/pretend play experiences to help the children relate to the sound system of our language. Explain the relationships in language the children can understand. You may want to provide props.

  Here are some examples:

  The letter B reminds me of a bouncing ball. As I bounce a ball on the floor, it says "b, b, b." The letter B makes the sound /b/. Let's all try to say it.

  The letter K is made with a lot of force. It reminds me of a kick. When you make the sound /k/, you need to use your tongue to kick out a lot of air. Let's make the sound /k/.

long *a*	You make a basket. Everyone says, "yeah."
short *a*	You eat something that tastes yucky.
b	Bounce a ball.
hard *c*	You have a bad cough. Cover your mouth and feel the cough.
soft *c*	Let air escape from a tire.
d	Play a drum with your hands. Now play it with your tongue.
long *e*	Make a siren sound.
short *e*	Lift a heavy weight above your head.
f	Light a firecracker. How does the fuse sound?
g	A little baby says, "googoogaga."
h	Blow hot air. Catch it in your hand.
long *i*	Show me your eye.
short *i*	Pick a worm off your arm.
j	Jump on a trampoline.
k	Kick out some air.
l	Sing the refrain from "Deck the Halls" (falalalala-lalalala).
m	How does pizza taste?
n	A shaking finger means "no."
long *o*	What do you say when you're surprised?
short *o*	Hug your stuffed animal and say the short *o* sound.
p	Pop your lips open like a balloon popping.
q	Make the /k/ sound and add long *u*.
r	Make a tight fist. Now make your tongue tight like your fist.
s	What does a rattlesnake say?
t	Tick like a clock.
long *u*	I'm pointing at "you."
short *u*	A punch in the stomach doesn't feel so good.
v	Make a sound like a motorboat.
w	Say, "double" and add long *u*.
x	Combine short *e*, /k/, and /s/.
y	You look sad. Why?
z	Here comes a bumblebee.
sh	The baby is sleeping. What does Mom say?
ch	Let's sneeze — ah-choo!
voiceless *th*	It's hot in here. Turn on the fan.
voiced *th*	Get that pesky fly!

- Explore how sounds are the same and different in place, manner, and voice. Compare the mouth posture pictures on pages 139 – 147 with the children.

- Associate the sound with its letter and alphabet sign, pages 13 – 17.

- Give the sound a label (e.g., /l/ — the singing sound, /g/ — the baby sound, /s/ — the snake sound).

Criterion for Moving to Phase Two

As mentioned in the Introduction, this program is based on the alphabet for practical reasons. A reasonable level of proficiency (75-80%) should be achieved before moving on to Phase Two of the program. Keep in mind that letter names are not equal in terms of ease of production and articulatory complexity. Some are much more difficult to make than others. Open vowels like short *o* and short *u* are easier than closed vowels like long *e* and short *i*. In typical development, children acquire consonants around the following ages (Prather et al, 1975):

Consonant	Key Word	Age in Years
m	man	2
n	nut	2
h	hat	2
p	pig	2
ng	king	2
f	fish	2-4
y	yes	2-4
k	kite	2-4
g	goat	2-4
d	dog	2-4
w	wig	2-8
b	ball	2-8
t	top	2-8
s	sun	3
l	log	3-4
r	rabbit	3-4
ch	chain	3-8
sh	shake	3-8
v	vest	4
z	zebra	4
zh	measure	4
voiceless th	think	4
voiced th	that	4
j	judge	4

Do not expect perfection from the children in the first cycles of Phase One. With some letter names, the goal may be to master only one feature of the sound (e.g., place, manner, or voice). Do not pass over any letter names because you feel the sound is developmentally too difficult. It is important to expose the children to all the sounds to stimulate their acquisition and not to be left with a few lingering error sounds at the end of the program.

Instructional Tools

Oral-Motor Mouth Postures

Pictures of lip and tongue placement for the oral-motor exercises in Phase One are provided on pages 27 – 28. Use the pictures for additional visual support when doing the exercises.

ABC Flash Cards

The flash cards in Phase One show a letter, and a word and picture containing a syllable that sounds like the letter name. The letter is the target; the word is the challenging context. (See pages 29 – 36.)

Supplemental Target List

Although Phase One targets sounds in isolation, it is important to challenge the children to use each sound in a more complex context. A challenging word is pictured on each ABC Flash Card. Use the supplemental list on page 37 for alternative challenging words or for additional practice.

Family Letter and Home Practice Materials

The Family Letter, page 38, briefly describes Phase One and suggests ways for the parents/caregivers to work with their child at home. Attach a copy of the ABC Flash Cards at the Sounds in Isolation level, pages 29 – 36, the Home Practice Log, page 39, and Home Practice Notes, page 40. Send these materials home with the children after the first session of the phase.

Phase Completion Certificate

Present the certificate, page 41, to the children when they complete Phase One.

Phase One Therapy

Materials
- Alphabet Mouth Postures, pages 139 – 147
- laminated set of ABC Flash Cards, pages 29 – 36, for use in therapy
- Oral-Motor Exercises – Mouth Postures, pages 27 – 28
- small, hand-held mirror for each child
- reinforcement activity, if needed, page 149
- Apraxia Group Response Form, page 151, or Apraxia Individual Response Form, page 153
- one set of ABC Flash Cards for each child, pages 29 – 36 , for practice at home
- one Family Letter, Home Practice Log, and Home Practice Notes for each child, pages 38 – 40
- Phase Completion Certificate for each child, page 41
- Supplemental Target List, page 37 (optional)

Session Sequence

❶ Gross Motor Warm-Up

Ask the children to perform a gross motor movement such as running in place, clapping, or doing jumping jacks while singing the ABC song. (See page 148 for additional gross motor movement activities.) Sing the song slowly with exaggerated articulation. Repeat the song and movement activity several times.

> "A, B, C, D, E, F, G,
> H, I, J, K, L-M-N-O-P,
> Q, R, S,
> T, U, V,
> W, X, Y, and Z.
> Now I know my ABCs.
> Next time won't you sing with me?"

❷ Oral-Motor Exercises

Ask the children to imitate the following lip and tongue exercises five times each. Display the mouth posture pictures, pages 27 – 28. Encourage the children to match the postures as they perform the exercises. Children may benefit from using their mirrors. Use your fingers to indicate the number of repetitions.

Lip Exercises
- Push your lips out and pull them back while you say, "ooo-eee."
- Make lots of slow and fast kisses.
- Squeeze your lips together while you say, "mmmm."

Tongue Exercises
- Stick out your tongue. Move the tip of your tongue from one corner of your mouth to the other.
- Make lots of slow and fast tongue clicks.
- Stick your tongue out, stretch it, and put it back in your mouth. Don't let your tongue touch your teeth.

❸ Alphabet Chant

Recite the alphabet in unison with the children using the Alphabet Chant found on pages 137 – 138. The chant requires the children to form the sign, say the letter name, and produce the associated sound(s). Use hand-over-hand assistance, if necessary, to form the signs. Show the Alphabet Mouth Posture pictures for added visual support in producing the sounds, pages 139 – 147.

Tips   • Encourage the children to watch your mouth for placement cues.

• Form the alphabet sign near your face to keep the children's attention focused on your face.

• Repeat the sound distinctly three times with a short pause between the repetitions. Prolong continuant sounds, repeating each prolongation three times.

• Present the long vowel sound first, then the short vowel sound.

• The letter C makes both the /k/ and the /s/ sound. Present both sounds.

• Present both the voiceless and voiced /th/ sounds.

• Develop a definite cadence to your alphabet review to provide prosodic support.

• Refer to a graphic representation of each letter (e.g., point to the letter on an alphabet chart, place a magnetic letter on a board, use an alphabet puzzle, write the letter on a chalkboard).

❹ Drill Sounds in Isolation

Drill is the most important factor for success in improving the intelligibility of children with apraxia. The children will come to expect drill as part of the program. Don't let them talk you out of it.

Practice the ABC Flash Cards at the Sounds in Isolation level. Include practice of the challenging context when the target is easily produced. Record the accuracy of each child's response (+/−) on the Apraxia Group Response Form, page 151, or the Apraxia Individual Response Form, page 153. Use the Supplemental Target List on page 37 for alternative words or for additional practice.

Tips   • Encourage precise articulation of each letter name.

• Establish a rapid pace.

• Elicit a high number of responses.

• Require three to five unison responses, followed by an individual response from each child.

• Cue sounds using the alphabet signs.

• Do not dwell on difficult sounds; provide a model and production cues, then go on.

• Elicit the target in a more complex context (the pictured word).

• If necessary, use a simple, quick, tangible reinforcer to keep the children on task. (See page 149.)

❺ Words of Increasing Length

Ask the children to repeat the following syllable groups until the whole utterance has been produced, cueing difficult sounds with the alphabet signs. Use hand gestures to establish an echoing routine. After practicing the whole utterance a few times, call on an individual child to use the utterance in response to the role play. Encourage dynamic expression.

- A - A B - A B Cs

  Role Play: Krista, we practiced saying the alphabet today. What is another name for the alphabet?

- I - I did - I did it!

  Role Play: Pablo, you make a goal at your soccer game. What do you say?

- Big - Big bad - Big bad wolf!

  Role Play: Jessie, Little Red Riding Hood didn't see Grandma in bed. Who was it?

- Give - Give me - Give me five!

  Role Play: Toby, you did a good job today. When I put my hand up like this, what does it mean?

- Way - Way to - Way to go!

  Role Play: Spencer, we all did a good job today. What can you tell the group?

❻ Song

Sing a familiar song with the children that uses letter names in the verse. Sing the song slowly with accentuated rhythm. Ask the children to use alphabet signs when they sing the letter names. A rhythmic, whole-body movement, such as swinging or clapping to the beat of the song, will facilitate sound production. Song suggestions include:

Old MacDonald

"Old MacDonald had a farm.
E-I-E-I-O!
And on his farm he had a horse (cow, pig, cat, dog, duck).
E-I-E-I-O!
With a neigh, neigh, here, and a neigh, neigh there.
Here a neigh, there a neigh, everywhere a neigh, neigh.
Old MacDonald had a farm.
E-I-E-I-O!"

BINGO

"There was a farmer had a dog and Bingo was his name-O.
B-I-N-G-O, B-I-N-G-O, B-I-N-G-O and Bingo was his name-O."
(Repeat.)

Mickey Mouse Club

"Mickey Mouse Club! Mickey Mouse Club!
Who's the leader of the club that's made for you and me?
M-I-C, K-E-Y, M-O-U-S-E.
Mickey Mouse! (Shout, "Mickey Mouse.")
Donald Duck! (Shout, "Donald Duck.")
Forever let us hold our banner high! (Shout, "High! High! High!")
Come along and sing a song and join our jamboree!
M-I-C, K-E-Y, M-O-U-S-E!"

7 Closure

Invite the parents/caregivers into the therapy room. Discuss the session and distribute the ABC Flash Cards, pages 29 – 36, Family Letter, page 38, Home Practice Log, page 39, and Home Practice Notes, page 40. Stress the importance of daily practice and remind the parents/caregivers to complete the home practice logs and notes. Suggest that the family sing the song used in therapy and read the books listed on the letter for additional practice and carryover. The songs and books should be presented slowly and with exaggerated rhythm and expression so the children have an opportunity to join in. Once the child is familiar with the song or book, the parent/caregiver should pause frequently to allow the child to fill in the letters and key words.

On the last day of the phase, present a Phase Completion Certificate to each child, page 41.

Oral Motor Exercises — Mouth Postures

Lip Exercises

Push your lips out and pull them back while you say, "ooo-eee."

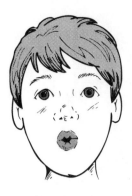 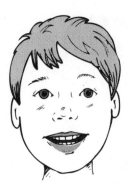

Make lots of slow and fast kisses.

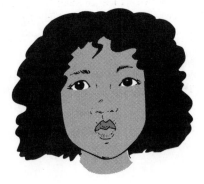

Squeeze your lips together while you say, "mmmm."

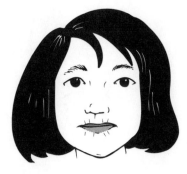

Oral Motor Exercises — Mouth Postures, continued

Tongue Exercises

Stick out your tongue. Move the tip of your tongue from one corner of your mouth to the other.

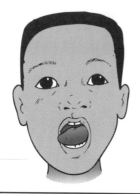 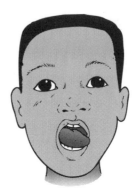

Make lots of slow and fast tongue clicks.

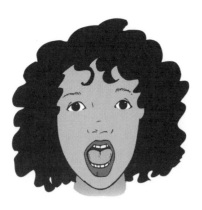 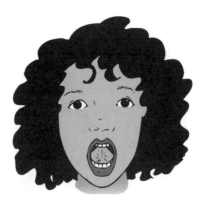

Stick your tongue out, stretch it, and put it back in your mouth. Don't let your tongue touch your teeth.

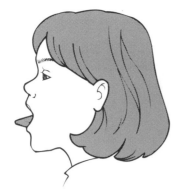 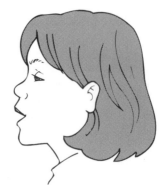

ABC Flash Cards

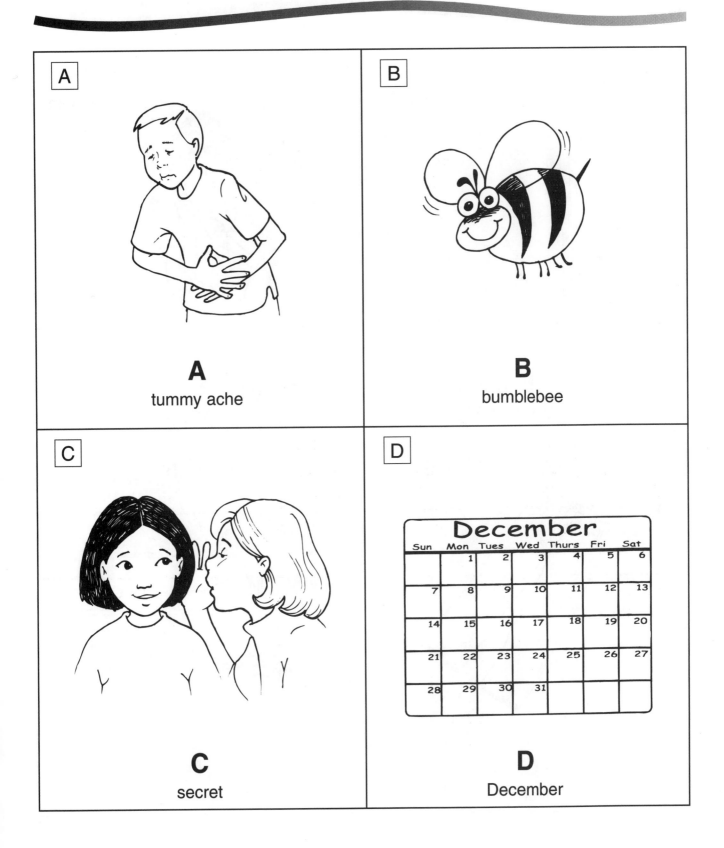

A

A

tummy ache

B

B

bumblebee

C

C

secret

D

D

December

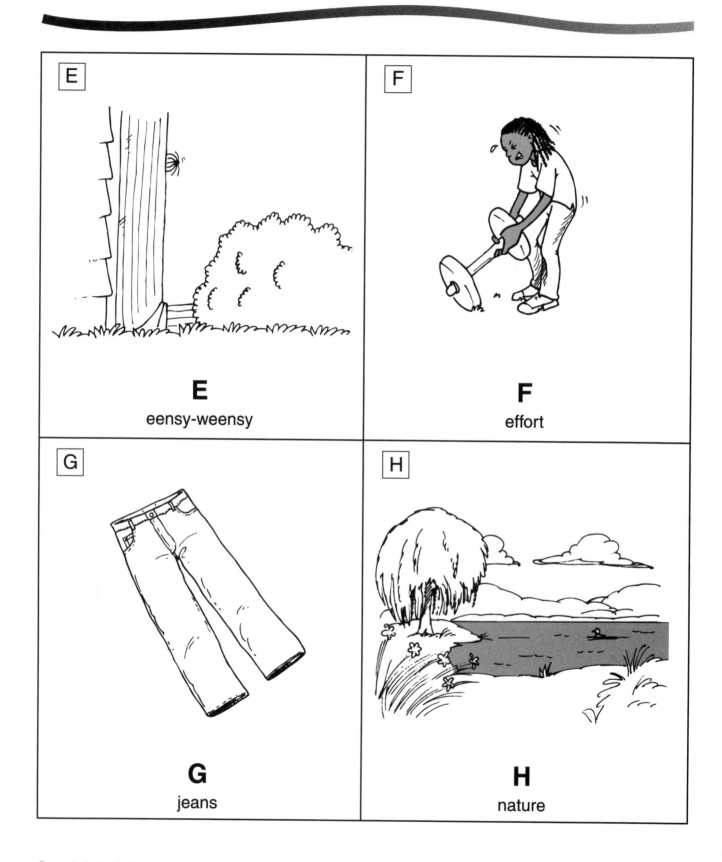

E

eensy-weensy

F

effort

G

jeans

H

nature

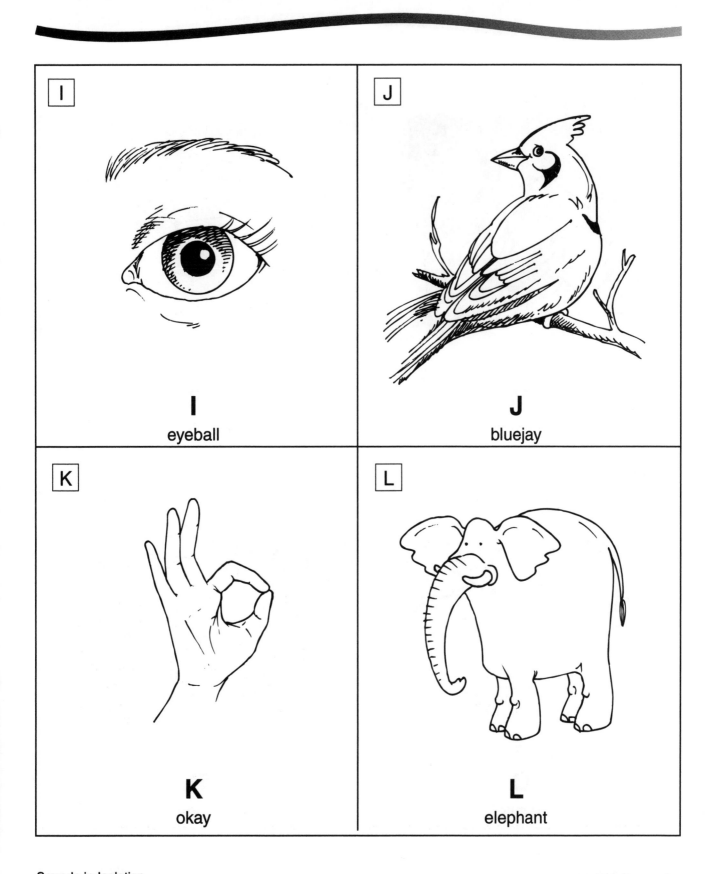

I

I
eyeball

J

J
bluejay

K

K
okay

L

L
elephant

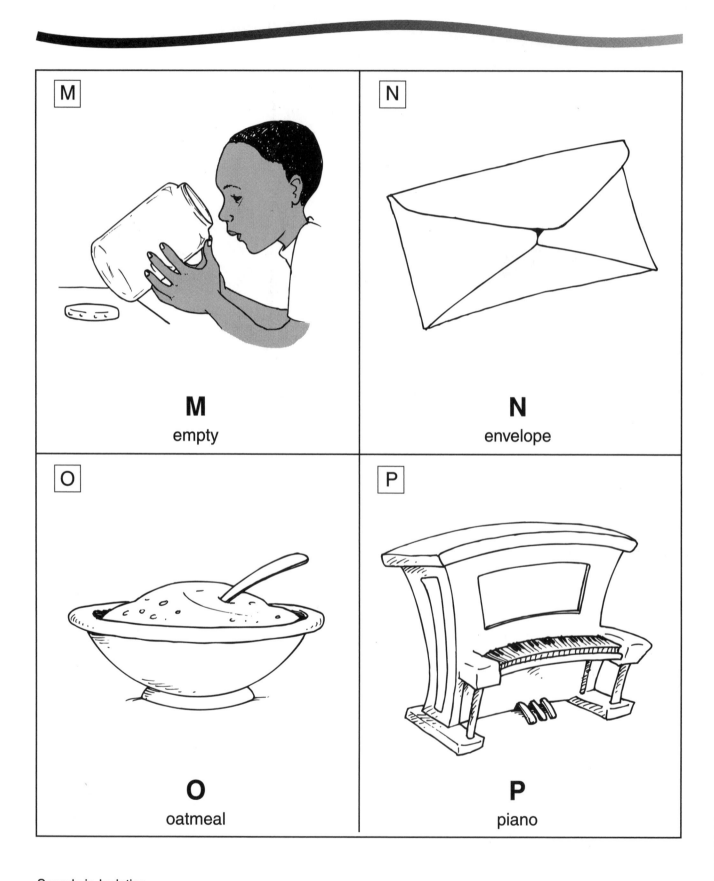

M
empty

N
envelope

O
oatmeal

P
piano

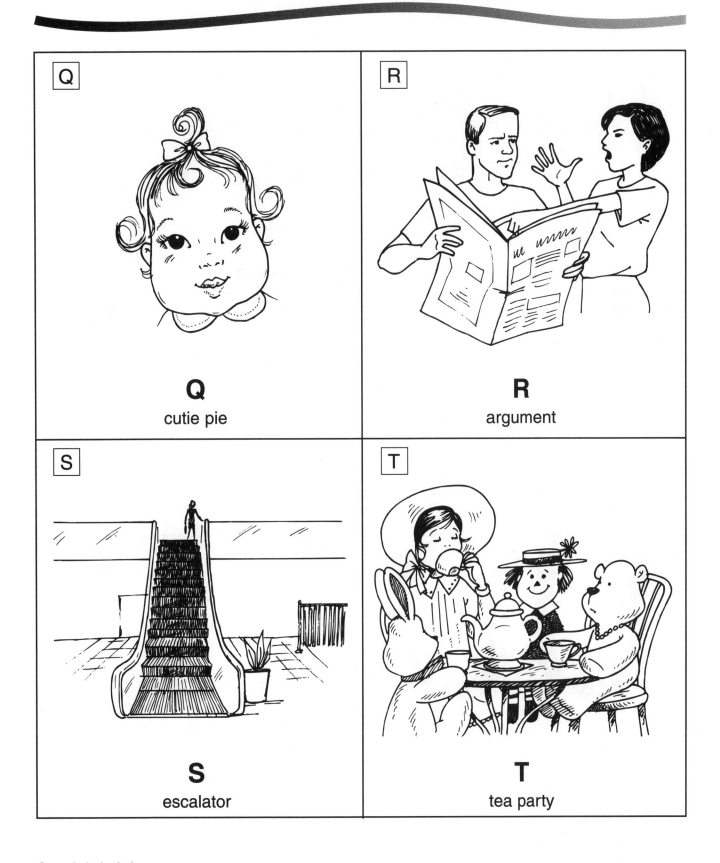

Q
cutie pie

R
argument

S
escalator

T
tea party

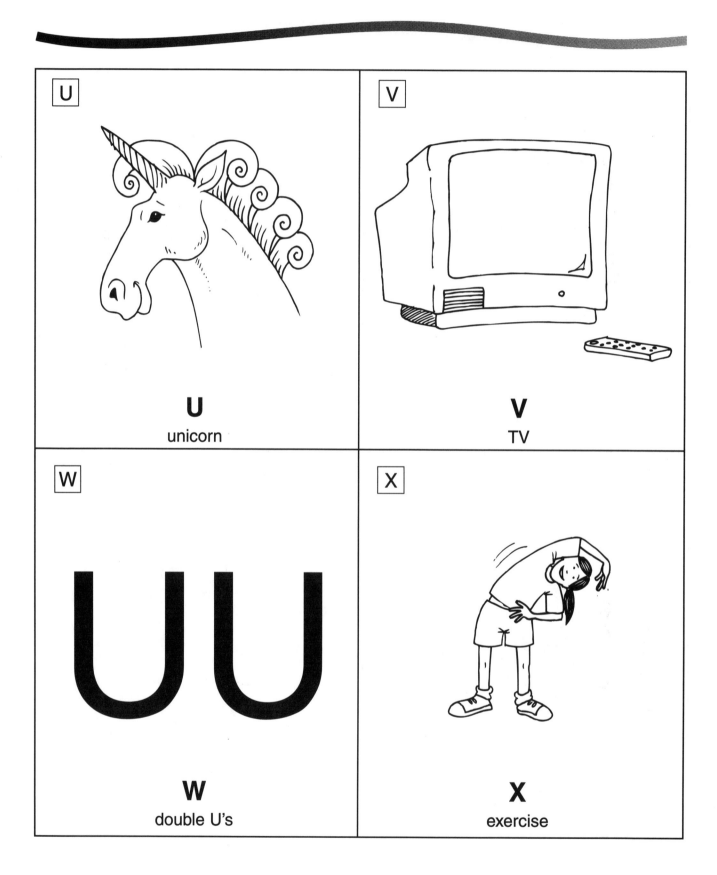

U **U** unicorn	V **V** TV
W **W** double U's	X **X** exercise

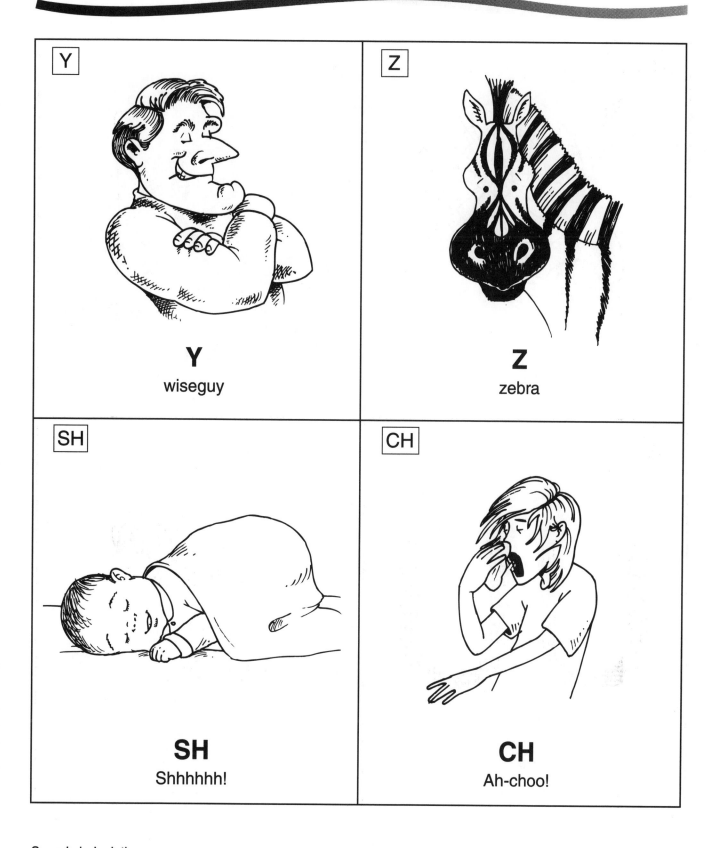

Y
wiseguy

Z
zebra

SH
Shhhhhh!

CH
Ah-choo!

35

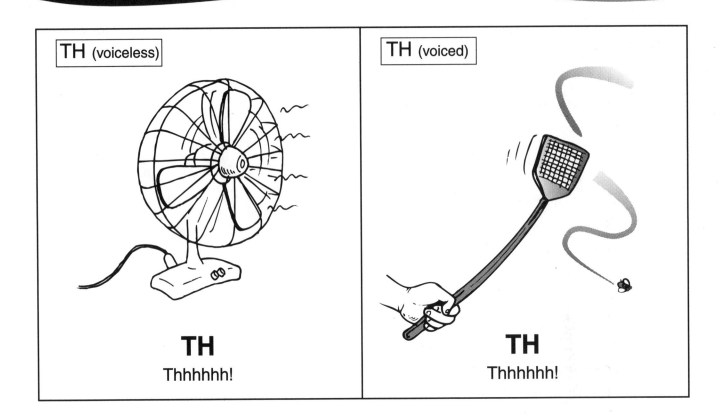

TH (voiceless)

TH
Thhhhhh!

TH (voiced)

TH
Thhhhhh!

Supplemental Target List

Use these words as alternatives to the pictured words on the ABC Flash Cards or for additional practice.

A — acorn, headache, ace, eight
B — Beanie Baby®, pork 'n' beans
C — scenery, loveseat, seesaw
D — teddy bear, lady, daddy, deep
E — eagle, eat, each, east, easy
F — left, leftover, Jeff, UFO, deaf
G — jeep, jeans, gee
H — Rachel, HBO, 4-H, VHS
I — eyelash, eyebrow, ice cream
J — jaywalk, Jake, Jane
K — suitcase, cane, cake, cape, cable
L — elbow pads, elevator, telephone
M — remember, Emma, M & M®s
N — enter, engine, energy
O — open, oatmeal, okay, oak, ocean
P — piano, peanut butter, peach, piece, peek, peel
Q — barbecue, porcupine, Q-tip®
R — argument, art class, arcade, archery
S — estimate, princess, waitress, pest, best
T — tea kettle, TV, teaspoon, tease, teacher
U — unicycle, uniform, ukulele
V — UV rays, Venus, vehicle, veal, veto
W — www.com, U-V-W
X — excellent, excitement, exit, exercise, experiment
Y — wipe, white, wire, while, wild, wide
Z — magazine, New Zealand
SH — shush, she, show, shy, shoe
CH — each, ouch, chew, chew toy
voiceless TH — thigh, eighth, oath, thin, thumb
voiced TH — they, the

Dear Family,

Today we began Phase One of your child's speech therapy program. It is called Sounds in Isolation. I will help your child say the letters of the alphabet in a precise and clear manner. We're starting with the alphabet for several reasons.

- You and your child are already familiar with the alphabet.
- It is something your child needs to know in the classroom.
- All but three consonant sounds in the English language (/ch/, /sh/, and /th/) are in the alphabet.

I'm sending home a set of ABC Flash Cards and home practice materials. The key to a successful speech program for your child is practice, and lots of it. Please practice the flash cards with your child every day. Remember to complete the Home Practice Log and a Home Practice Note every time you drill the ABC Flash Cards with your child.

Encourage your child to watch your mouth when you practice. Do not expect your child to pronounce all alphabet letters perfectly at first. Some letter names are much more difficult to say than others. Many of the pictured words will be challenging. Stress the syllable that makes the sound of the letter name, like "bee" in the word *bumblebee*. These words will give your child extra practice after he/she can easily say the sound by itself.

Besides drilling the flash cards, you can practice the alphabet in other ways. You can sing songs that spell words and/or read alphabet books. Here are a few suggestions:

Songs
- *Old MacDonald*
- *BINGO*
- *Mickey Mouse Club*

Books
- *Chicka Chicka ABC* by Bill Martin Jr and John Archambault
- *Dr. Seuss's ABC* by Dr. Seuss
- *Ape in a Cape* by Fritz Eichenberg
- *Alphabatics* by Suse MacDonald

Thank you for your support. Please call if you have questions or concerns. You are always invited to observe your child in therapy.

Sincerely,

_____

Speech-Language Pathologist

_____

Phone

Home Practice Log

Child: _____ Speech-Language Pathologist: _____

Parent/Caregiver: Please practice the ABC Flash Cards at the Sounds in Isolation level with your child daily (at least 5 days per week). Mark a **+** in the box when your child pronounces the letter name correctly; mark a **–** in the box when your child incorrectly pronounces the letter name. Record the total number of correct responses in the box at the bottom of the column. Please return this log when completed or at the end of this phase. Thanks!

Date															
A															
B															
C															
D															
E															
F															
G															
H															
I															
J															
K															
L															
M															
N															
O															
P															
Q															
R															
S															
T															
U															
V															
W															
X															
Y															
Z															
SH															
CH															
TH (voiceless)															
TH (voiced)															
Total Correct															

Sounds in Isolation
Just for Kids: Apraxia

Home Practice Notes

Parent/Caregiver: Please complete a Home Practice Note after each practice session with your child. Record the number of correct responses from the Home Practice Log in the space provided. Ask your child to return the note to speech therapy for a reward. Thanks!

We practiced the ABC Flash Cards at the Sounds in Isolation level today.

_____ pronounced _____ letter names correctly!
Child   *number*

_____   _____
Parent/Caregiver Signature   *Date*

(Please return to Speech-Language Therapy.)   ☐ Send more notes.

We practiced the ABC Flash Cards at the Sounds in Isolation level today.

_____ pronounced _____ letter names correctly!
Child   *number*

_____   _____
Parent/Caregiver Signature   *Date*

(Please return to Speech-Language Therapy.)   ☐ Send more notes.

We practiced the ABC Flash Cards at the Sounds in Isolation level today.

_____ pronounced _____ letter names correctly!
Child   *number*

_____   _____
Parent/Caregiver Signature   *Date*

(Please return to Speech-Language Therapy.)   ☐ Send more notes.

We practiced the ABC Flash Cards at the Sounds in Isolation level today.

_____ pronounced _____ letter names correctly!
Child   *number*

_____   _____
Parent/Caregiver Signature   *Date*

(Please return to Speech-Language Therapy.)   ☐ Send more notes.

We practiced the ABC Flash Cards at the Sounds in Isolation level today.

_____ pronounced _____ letter names correctly!
Child   *number*

_____   _____
Parent/Caregiver Signature   *Date*

(Please return to Speech-Language Therapy.)   ☐ Send more notes.

A • B • C • D • E • F • G • H • I • J • K • L • M •

Sounds in Isolation

This is to certify that

_____

has successfully completed

Phase One of the

Apraxia Therapy Program.

Speech-Language Pathologist

_____
Date

U • T • S • R • Q • P • O • N •
Z • Y • X • W • V •

Phase Completion Certificate
Just for Kids: Apraxia

C-V-C Words
Phase Two

Rationale

C-V-C Words: Phase Two begins the focus on movement transitions. Speech is not merely a series of sounds, but rather sounds blended together. Children with apraxia of speech can often produce sounds in isolation correctly, but break down when sounds are combined into words. As the linguistic and phonetic complexity of an utterance increases, intelligibility decreases. Errors in articulation include:

- vowel distortions and substitutions
- consonant deletions, substitutions, and transpositions
- blend reductions
- syllable deletions and assimilations

Sounds in Isolation: Phase One helped the children build sound-letter associations. The first phase of the program stressed the letter, a more familiar concept to young children than sounds, and related the letter to its associated sound. In Phase Two, sounds are stressed in functional, high frequency C-V-C words. (Although the sounds associated with the letters Q and X are technically blends – /kw/ and /ks/ respectively – they have been included for consistency and to avoid confusing the children.)

It is essential in apraxia therapy to move quickly from production of sounds in isolation to the production of sound sequences. It is in moving from one sound to another that these children have the greatest difficulty, requiring intensive practice to habituate the transitions. Nonsense syllables and nonsense words are not used in this program. It is more functional and efficient to move from sounds in isolation to carefully controlled real words so that children have words they can use in their daily interactions. The power of successful communication is the best motivator of all.

Strategies

Sound combinations are difficult for children with apraxia of speech. Their ability to execute and remember the movements for connected speech is severely limited. The following strategies will facilitate success in Phase Two.

- Continue to emphasize the visual channel. The children need to watch your face, see the letters, match mouth postures, watch each other, and use a mirror.

- Encourage the children to feel the changes in air, sound, and movement within words. For example:
  - Place the child's hand on the throat in front of the larynx to feel the vibration.
  - Have the child close her eyes and stop voicing to concentrate on articulatory movements.

- Cue the sound sequences with the alphabet signs, pages 13 – 17. Encourage the children to use the signs too.

- Help the children understand that words are made up of individual sounds by associating each sound with a different colored block or mouth posture picture (pages 139 – 147). Always blend the individual sounds into the target word.

- Use forward or backward chaining to combine the sounds in the target word. For example:

    Forward chaining:
    b – be – bed

    Backward chaining:
    t – at – cat

- Success breeds success. Set up the tasks so the children are successful. Simultaneous productions give the children maximal cues. Move to mouth posture cues, then imitation, and finally an imposed delay (Strand, 1994).

- Stress "careful" speech. Encourage the child to take the responsibility to slow down, use precise articulation, and monitor his speech.

- Put responsibility on the children for remembering a sound or a word and then using it in a more complex context.

- Have the children sit on a large ball during therapy. This allows them to expend excess energy and enhances overall stability and sensory integration. The ball should "fit" the child, allowing her to place her feet on the floor. It is best to have the children sit away from the table so they do not lean on the table for support.

- Challenge the children to use target words in short phrases, especially words that are easily produced. A suggested phrase is provided on the ABC Flash Cards (pages 52 – 59).

- A slower rate of speech will give the children the additional time needed to plan, execute, and sequence the sounds in words.

Criterion for Moving to Phase Three

Unlike articulation and phonological processes programs, the target for *C-V-C Words: Phase Two* is not a sound or a process (or a letter of the alphabet). It is the movement transitions required to produce the C-V-C word. Therefore, when judging the accuracy of a response in Phase Two, consider the whole word. All of the sounds in the word must be correct. A 75-80% proficiency level should be achieved before moving to Phase Three of the program. Since children with apraxia do not acquire speech in the same manner as other children, do not delete any words based on developmental acquisition norms. Keep in mind that it is not the sound, but the sequencing of sounds that causes their difficulty. You do not want one or two sound patterns to be deficient at the end of the program because of a lack of exposure.

Instructional Tools

Oral-Motor Mouth Postures

Pictures of lip and tongue placement for the oral-motor exercises in Phase Two are provided on pages 50 – 51. Use the pictures for additional visual support when doing the exercises.

ABC Flash Cards

The flash cards in Phase Two show a C-V-C word and picture, and a phrase or sentence containing the C-V-C word. The C-V-C word is the target; the phrase or sentence is the challenging context. (See pages 52 – 59.)

Supplemental Target List

A supplemental list of C-V-C words is provided on page 60. Use this list for alternative words or additional practice.

Family Letter and Home Practice Materials

The Family Letter, page 61, briefly describes Phase Two and suggests ways for the parents/ caregivers to work with their child at home. Attach a copy of the ABC Flash Cards at the C-V-C Words level, pages 52 – 59, the Home Practice Log, page 62, and Home Practice Notes, page 63. Send these materials home with the children after the first session of the phase.

Phase Completion Certificate

Present the certificate, page 64, to the children when they complete Phase Two.

Phase Two Therapy

Materials
- Alphabet Mouth Postures, pages 139 – 147
- laminated set of ABC Flash Cards, pages 52 – 59, for use in therapy
- Oral-Motor Exercises – Mouth Postures, pages 50 – 51
- small, hand-held mirror for each child
- reinforcement activity, if needed, page 149
- Apraxia Group Response Form, page 151, or Apraxia Individual Response Form, page 153
- one set of ABC Flash Cards for each child, pages 52 – 59, for practice at home
- one Family Letter, Home Practice Log, and Home Practice Notes for each child, pages 61 – 63
- Phase Completion Certificate for each child, page 64
- Supplemental Target List, page 60 (optional)

Session Sequence

❶ Gross Motor Warm-Up

Ask the children to perform a gross motor movement such as running in place, clapping, or doing jumping jacks while singing the ABC song. (See page 148 for additional gross motor movement activities.) Sing the song slowly with exaggerated articulation. Repeat the song and movement activity several times.

> "A, B, C, D, E, F, G,
> H, I, J, K, L-M-N-O-P,
> Q, R, S,
> T, U, V,
> W, X, Y, and Z.
> Now I know my ABCs.
> Next time won't you sing with me?"

❷ Oral-Motor Exercises

Ask the children to imitate the following lip and tongue exercises five times each. Display the mouth posture pictures on pages 50 – 51, encouraging the children to match the postures as they perform the exercises. Children may benefit from using their mirrors. Use your fingers to indicate the number of repetitions.

Lip Exercises
- Rub and then firmly tap around your lips.

- Make the motor sound for three to five seconds.

- Lift one corner of your lips to show the molars on that side of your mouth. Now do the same on the other side.

Tongue Exercises
- Rub your bottom lip with your tongue, then your top lip.

- Try to poke your tongue through your right cheek, then your left cheek.

- Stick your tongue out, stretch it, and put it back in your mouth. Don't let your tongue touch your teeth.

❸ Alphabet Chant

Recite the alphabet in unison with the children using the Alphabet Chant found on pages 137 – 138. The chant requires the children to form the sign, say the letter name, and produce the associated sound(s). Use hand-over-hand assistance, if necessary, to form the signs. Show the Alphabet Mouth Posture pictures for added visual support in producing the sounds, pages 139 – 147.

Tips   • Encourage the children to watch your mouth for placement cues.

• Form the alphabet sign near your face to keep the children's attention focused on your face.

• Repeat the sound distinctly three times with a short pause between the repetitions. Prolong continuant sounds, repeating each prolongation three times.

• Present the long vowel sound first, then the short vowel sound.

• The letter C makes the /k/ and the /s/ sound. Present both sounds.

• Present both the voiceless and voiced /th/ sounds.

• Develop a definite cadence to your alphabet review to provide prosodic support.

• Refer to a graphic representation of each letter (e.g., point to the letter on an alphabet chart, place a magnetic letter on a board, use an alphabet puzzle, write the letter on a chalkboard).

❹ Drill C-V-C Words

Drill is the most important factor for success in improving the intelligibility of children with apraxia. The children will come to expect drill as part of the program. Don't let them talk you out of it.

Practice the ABC Flash Cards at the C-V-C Words level. Include practice of the challenging context when the target is easily produced. Record the accuracy of each child's response (+/−) on the Apraxia Group Response Form, page 151, or the Apraxia Individual Response Form, page 153. Use the Supplemental Target List on page 60 for alternative words or for additional practice.

Tips   • Encourage correct articulation of all sounds in the word.

• Stretch out the sounds in the words, especially the vowels, to give the children time to move to the next sound.

• Establish a rapid pace.

• Elicit a high number of responses.

• Require three to five unison responses, followed by an individual response from each child.

• Cue sounds using the alphabet signs.

• Do not dwell on difficult words. Provide a model and production cues, then go on.

- Elicit the target word in a more complex context (the suggested phrase).

- If necessary, use a simple, quick, tangible reinforcer to keep the children on task. (See page 149.)

❺ Words of Increasing Length

Ask the children to repeat the following syllable groups until the whole utterance has been produced, cueing difficult sounds with the alphabet signs. Use hand gestures to establish an echoing routine. After practicing the whole utterance a few times, call on an individual child to use the utterance in response to the role play. Encourage dynamic expression.

- Oh - Oh me - Oh me, oh - Oh me, oh my!

  Role Play: Kristina, you spilled your drink. What does Mom say?

- Read (red) - Ready - Ready, set - Ready, set, go!

  Role Play: Joey, you are at the start of a race. What do you say?

- Oops - Oopsy - Oopsy dai - Oopsy daisy!

  Role Play: Maria, something fell. What do you say?

- Fe - Fe fi - Fe fi fo - Fe fi fo fum!

  Role Play: Raul, the giant in Jack and the Beanstalk smells the boy. What does he say?

- Hip - Hip hip - Hip hip hur - Hip hip hurray!

  Role Play: Lacey, you won a prize! What do you say?

❻ Song

Sing a familiar song with the children that repeats common C-V-C words. Sing the song slowly with accentuated rhythm. Cue the first sound in key words with the alphabet signs. A rhythmic, whole-body movement, such as swinging or clapping to the beat of the song, will facilitate word production. Song suggestions include:

Jack and Jill

"Jack and Jill went up the hill
To fetch a pail of water.
Jack fell down and broke his crown,
And Jill came tumbling after.
Up Jack got and home he ran
As fast as he could caper.
There his mother bound his head
With vinegar and brown paper."

This Old Man

"This old man, he played one.
He played knick-knack on my thumb.

CHORUS: With a knick-knack, paddy whack,
                  Give a dog a bone.
                  This old man came rolling home.

"This old man, he played two.
He played knick-knack on my shoe. (CHORUS)

"This old man, he played three.
He played knick-knack on my knee. (CHORUS)

"This old man, he played four.
He played knick-knack on my door. (CHORUS)

"This old man, he played five.
He played knick-knack on my hive. (CHORUS)

"This old man, he played six.
He played knick-knack on my sticks. (CHORUS)

"This old man, he played seven.
He played knick-knack up in heaven. (CHORUS)

"This old man, he played eight.
He played knick-knack on my gate. (CHORUS)

"This old man, he played nine.
He played knick-knack on my line. (CHORUS)

"This old man, he played ten.
He played knick-knack on my hen. (CHORUS)"

Take Me Out to the Ball Game

"Take me out to the ball game.
Take me out with the crowd.
Buy me some peanuts and Cracker Jacks®.
I don't care if I ever get back.
Let me root, root, root for the home team.
If they don't win it's a shame.
For it's one, two, three strikes, you're out
At the old ball game."

7 Closure

Invite the parents/caregivers into the therapy room. Discuss the session and distribute the ABC Flash Cards, pages 52 – 59, Family Letter, page 61, Home Practice Log, page 62, and Home Practice Notes, page 63. Stress the importance of daily practice and remind the parents/caregivers to complete the home practice logs and notes. Suggest that the family sing the song used in therapy and read the books listed on the letter for additional practice and carryover. The songs and books should be presented slowly and with exaggerated rhythm and expression so the children have an opportunity to join in. Once the child is familiar with the song or book, the parent/caregiver should pause frequently to allow the child to fill in the rhyming words.

On the last day of the phase, present a Phase Completion Certificate to each child, page 64.

Oral-Motor Exercises — Mouth Postures

Lip Exercises

Rub, then firmly tap around your lips.

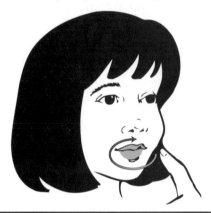 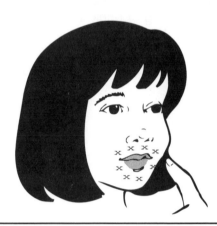

Make the motor sound for three to five seconds.

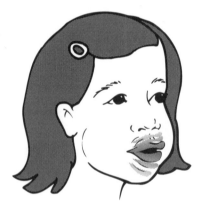

Lift one corner of your lips to show the molars on that side of your mouth. Now do the same on the other side.

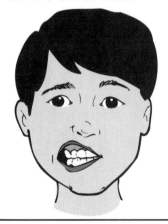 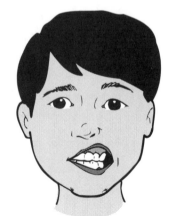

Oral Motor Exercises — Mouth Postures, continued

Tongue Exercises

Rub your bottom lip with your tongue, then your top lip.

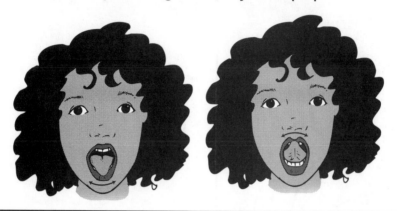

Try to poke your tongue through your right cheek, then your left cheek.

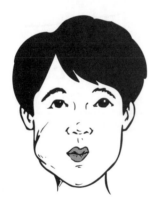 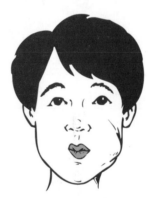

Stick your tongue out, stretch it, and put it back in your mouth. Don't let your tongue touch your teeth.

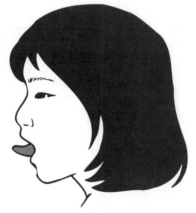

ABC Flash Cards

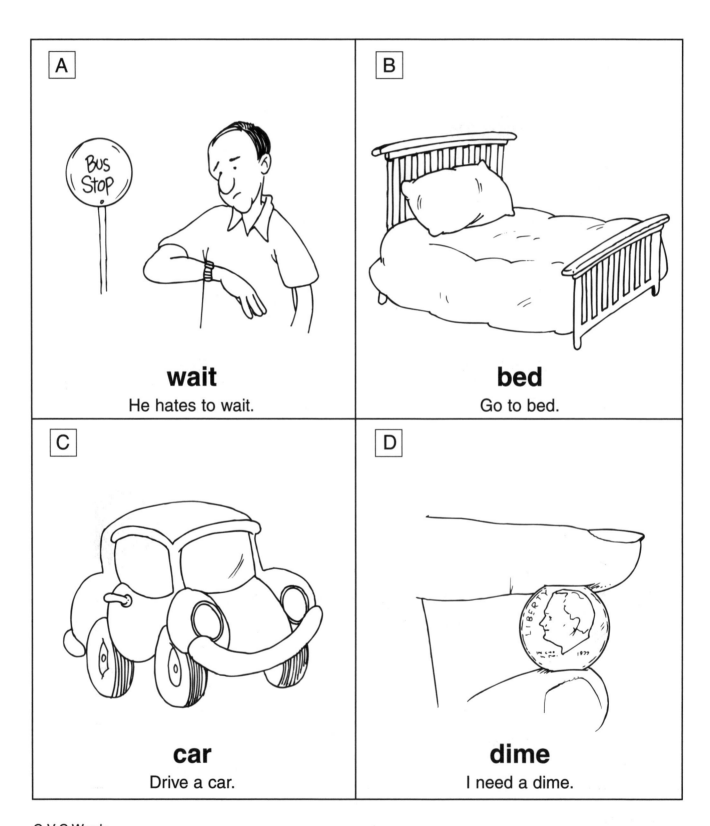

A

wait

He hates to wait.

B

bed

Go to bed.

C

car

Drive a car.

D

dime

I need a dime.

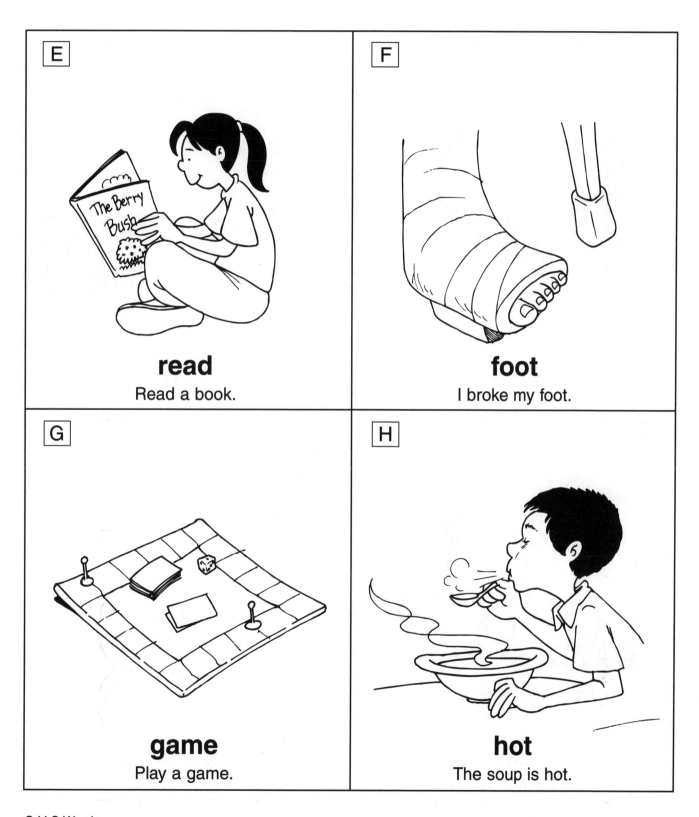

E

read

Read a book.

F

foot

I broke my foot.

G

game

Play a game.

H

hot

The soup is hot.

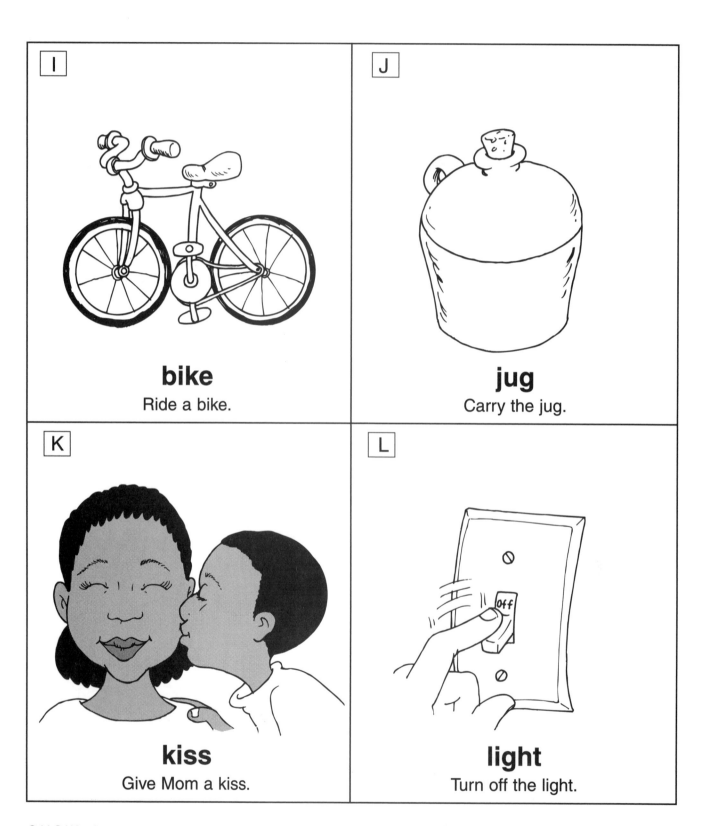

I

bike
Ride a bike.

J

jug
Carry the jug.

K

kiss
Give Mom a kiss.

L

light
Turn off the light.

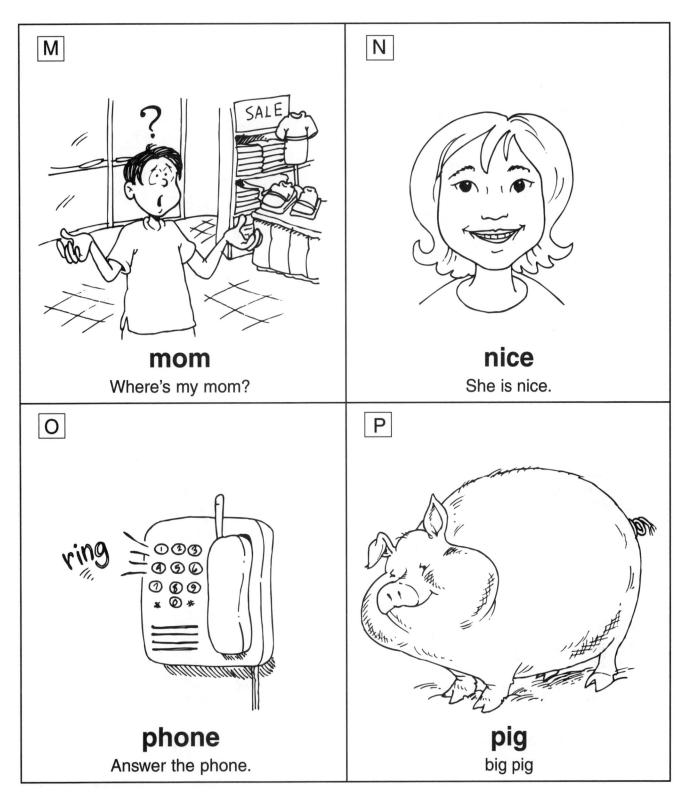

M

mom
Where's my mom?

N

nice
She is nice.

O

phone
Answer the phone.

P

pig
big pig

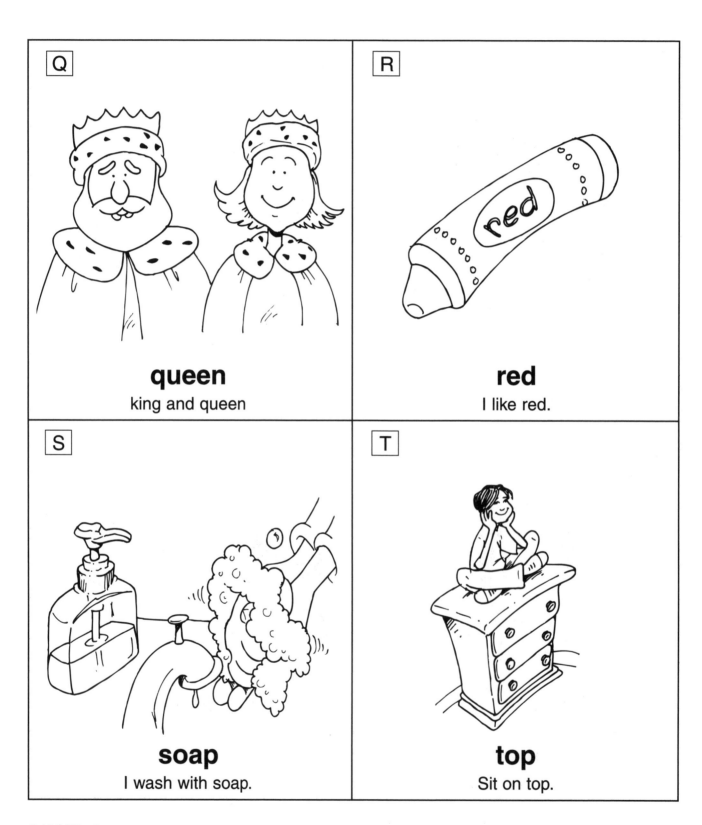

Q

queen
king and queen

R

red
I like red.

S

soap
I wash with soap.

T

top
Sit on top.

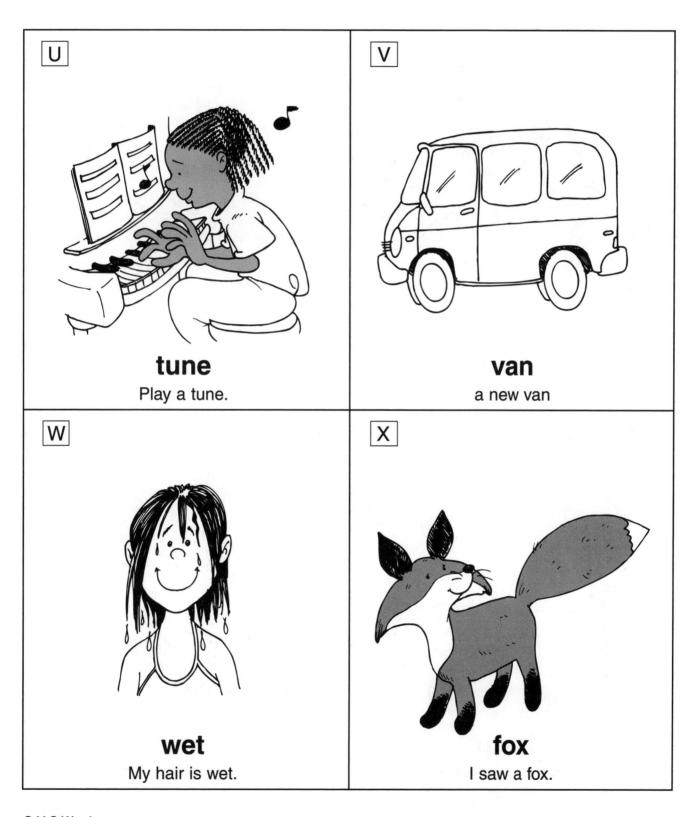

U

tune

Play a tune.

V

van

a new van

W

wet

My hair is wet.

X

fox

I saw a fox.

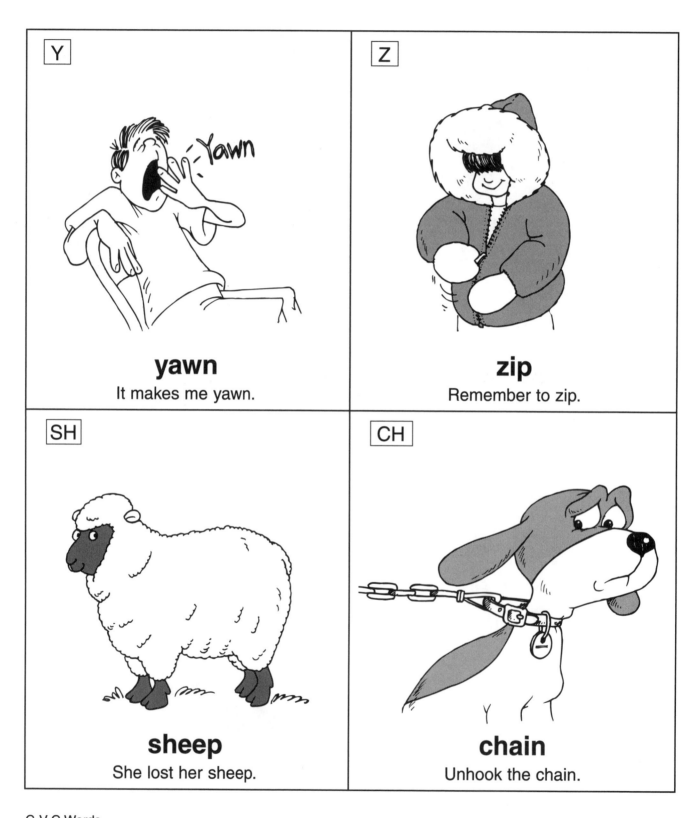

Y

yawn

It makes me yawn.

Z

zip

Remember to zip.

SH

sheep

She lost her sheep.

CH

chain

Unhook the chain.

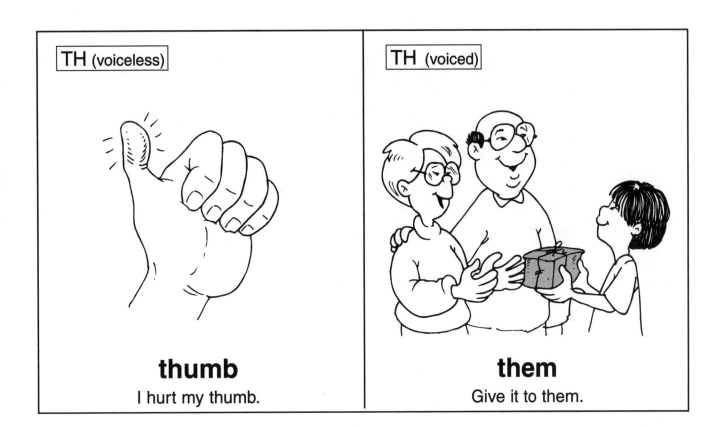

TH (voiceless)

thumb

I hurt my thumb.

TH (voiced)

them

Give it to them.

Supplemental Target List

Use these words as alternatives for the C-V-C words on the ABC Flash Cards or for additional practice.

A — cane, rain, tape, late, gate

B — bat, ball, bake, bike, big, bug, bear, boot, bone

C — can, cake, cat, cape, cave, cane, cap, comb

D — dog, door, date, duck, dash, deer, deep

E — seat, bean, seed, feet, teen, peek

F — five, fun, food, face, fall, fur, phone, feel, fan

G — good, goat, gate, gum, goose, gas, give

H — head, hide, hill, hot, house, hoop, hut

I — kite, right, bite, pipe, rhyme, dime, dice

J — jeep, judge, juice, jam, jet, job

K — kite, keep, king, kick, kit, kid

L — love, lake, lid, lamb, lip, leaf, look, leg, log

M — meat, mop, make, mud, moon, mouse, map, man

N — nice, nail, name, neck, nose, note, knock, near, night

O — boat, coat, cone, comb, loaf, rope, joke

P — pet, pan, pen, peach, pack, pig, pop, pear, pup

Q — quack, quake, quiz, quit, quick

R — read, write, rain, rut, rush, rat, rake, run, rug, rope

S — seed, sack, sit, sad, soup, sock, song, sun, sign

T — ten, tap, tall, time, tame, team, tag, tail

U — duke, dune, cube, suit, cute

V — veil, vase, vet, vote, vine, voice

W— weed, wag, wait, wood, web, wish

X — box, fix, rocks, mix, wax, locks

Y — year, yell, yes, young, yet

Z — zoom, zig, zag, zone

SH — ship, shout, shop, shape, sheet, shut, shell, shine

CH — chop, chair, chin, cheese, chip, cheek

voiceless TH — thin, thick, thing, thief, thud

voiced TH — this, that, them, there, these, those

Home Practice Notes

Parent/Caregiver: Please complete a Home Practice Note after each practice session with your child. Record the number of correct responses from the Home Practice Log in the space provided. Ask your child to return the note to speech therapy for a reward. Thanks!

We practiced the ABC Flash Cards at the C-V-C Words level today.

_____ pronounced _____ words correctly!
Child   number

_____   _____
Parent/Caregiver Signature   Date

(Please return to Speech-Language Therapy.)   ☐ Send more notes.

We practiced the ABC Flash Cards at the C-V-C Words level today.

_____ pronounced _____ words correctly!
Child   number

_____   _____
Parent/Caregiver Signature   Date

(Please return to Speech-Language Therapy.)   ☐ Send more notes.

We practiced the ABC Flash Cards at the C-V-C Words level today.

_____ pronounced _____ words correctly!
Child   number

_____   _____
Parent/Caregiver Signature   Date

(Please return to Speech-Language Therapy.)   ☐ Send more notes.

We practiced the ABC Flash Cards at the C-V-C Words level today.

_____ pronounced _____ words correctly!
Child   number

_____   _____
Parent/Caregiver Signature   Date

(Please return to Speech-Language Therapy.)   ☐ Send more notes.

We practiced the ABC Flash Cards at the C-V-C Words level today.

_____ pronounced _____ words correctly!
Child   number

_____   _____
Parent/Caregiver Signature   Date

(Please return to Speech-Language Therapy.)   ☐ Send more notes.

hot • bike • jug • kiss • light

zip • wait • bed • car • dime • read • foot • game

yawn • fox • wet • van • tune • top

soap • red • queen • pig • phone • nice • mom

C-V-C Words

This is to certify that

_____

has successfully completed

Phase Two of the

Apraxia Therapy Program.

_____
Speech-Language Pathologist

_____
Date

Phase Completion Certificate
Just for Kids: Apraxia

Multisyllabic Words
Phase Three

Rationale

Multisyllabic Words: Phase Three addresses movement transitions within two- to four-syllable words. Children with apraxia have difficulty shifting from one movement pattern to another in multisyllabic words. The following errors are often observed:

- deleting a syllable (*nana* for *banana*)
- transposing syllables (*bufferty* for *butterfly*)
- adding extra syllables (*fingerganail* for *fingernail*)
- repeating sounds (*dandy dar* for *candy bar*)
- deleting sounds (*Poicle* for *Popsicle®*)

At this point in therapy, the children should have a good knowledge of the structure of the program and what is expected of them. Sessions should move smoothly, with few directions from you and a lot of practice time. The children should be observing your visual and facial cues and forming most of the alphabet signs independently. Sometimes a child may need extra guidance. Sit close to this child and provide additional nonverbal feedback to keep him on task and to not hold the other children back.

Strategies

Sequenced syllable productions can be very confusing for children with apraxia. Provide as much structure as needed to set the children up for success. The following strategies will facilitate production:

- Signal the first sound in each syllable with the alphabet sign. For children who tend to delete final sounds, also signal the final sound in each syllable of the word.

- Ask the children to count the number of syllables in the multisyllabic word before producing it.

- Clap (or stomp, tap, snap, etc.) the syllables as you say them. Encourage the children to do the same.

- Make up cards with two, three, and four stickers on them. Choose the appropriate card and ask the children to point to a sticker on the card as they say each syllable.

- Find the little word within the big word and stress it while saying the word. For example, *mom* in *thermometer* and *sick* in *Popsicle®*.

- Overemphasize the stressed syllable in the multisyllabic word.

- Use forward and backward chaining. For example:

    Forward chaining:
    bum - bumble - bumblebee

    Backward chaining:
    cane - dycane - candy cane

- Model a slightly slower rate of production. The children will follow your lead.

- Challenge the children to use easily produced multisyllabic words in the carrier phrases suggested on the ABC Flash Cards.

Criterion for Moving to Phase Four

As in *C-V-C Words: Phase Two*, all sounds in the multisyllabic word must be correct for it to be scored as a correct response. Expect the children to achieve a 75-80% accuracy level before moving to Phase Four. If possible, provide additional individual therapy to a child who is lagging behind or solicit the help of a volunteer or aide.

Instructional Tools

Oral-Motor Mouth Postures

Pictures of lip and tongue placement for the oral-motor exercises in Phase Three are provided on pages 71 – 72. Use the pictures for additional visual support when doing the exercises.

ABC Flash Cards

The flash cards in Phase Three show a multisyllabic word and picture, and a carrier phrase (e.g., "I see, I have, I need, I want, I found"). The multisyllabic word is the target; the carrier phrase is the challenging context. (See pages 73 – 80.)

Supplemental Target List

A supplemental list of multisyllabic words is provided on page 81. Use this list for alternative words or additional practice.

Family Letter and Home Practice Materials

The Family Letter, page 82, briefly describes Phase Three and suggests ways for the parents/ caregivers to work with their child at home. Attach a copy of the ABC Flash Cards at the Multisyllabic Words level, pages 73 – 80, the Home Practice Log, page 83, and Home Practice Notes, page 84.   Send these materials home with the children after the first session of the phase.

Phase Completion Certificate

Present the certificate, page 85, to the children when they complete Phase Three.

Phase Three Therapy

Materials
- Alphabet Mouth Postures, pages 139 – 147
- laminated set of ABC Flash Cards, pages 73 – 80, for use in therapy
- Oral-Motor Exercises – Mouth Postures, pages 71 – 72
- small, hand-held mirror for each child
- reinforcement activity, if needed, page 149
- Apraxia Group Response Form, page 151, or Apraxia Individual Response Form, page 153
- one set of ABC Flash Cards for each child, pages 73 – 80, for practice at home
- one Family Letter, Home Practice Log, and Home Practice Notes for each child, pages 82 – 84
- Phase Completion Certificate for each child, page 85
- Supplemental Target List, page 81 (optional)

Session Sequence

❶ Gross Motor Warm-Up

Ask the children to perform a gross motor movement such as running in place, clapping, or doing jumping jacks while singing the ABC song. (See page 148 for additional gross motor movement activities.) Sing the song slowly with exaggerated articulation. Repeat the song and movement activity several times.

"A, B, C, D, E, F, G,
H, I, J, K, L-M-N-O-P,
Q, R, S,
T, U, V,
W, X, Y, and Z.
Now I know my ABCs.
Next time won't you sing with me?"

❷ Oral-Motor Exercises

Ask the children to imitate the following lip and tongue exercises five times each. Display the mouth posture pictures on pages 71 – 72, encouraging the children to match the postures as they perform the exercises. Children may benefit from using their mirrors. Use your fingers to indicate the number of repetitions.

Lip Exercises
- Kiss the palm of your hand. Then blow a kiss.

- Make slow lip pops, then fast ones.

- Hide your upper lip with your lower lip. Then hide your lower lip with your upper lip.

Tongue Exercises
- Point your tongue toward your chin. Then move it toward your nose. Try to stretch your tongue a little farther each time.

- Use your tongue tip to circle your lips. Go in one direction and then the other. Don't miss the corners of your lips.

- Curl up the sides of your tongue. Then move your tongue in and out of your mouth.

❸ Alphabet Chant

Recite the alphabet in unison with the children using the Alphabet Chant found on pages 137 – 138. The chant requires the children to form the sign, say the letter name, and produce the associated sound(s). Use hand-over-hand assistance, if necessary, to form the signs. Show the Alphabet Mouth Posture pictures for added visual support in producing the sounds, pages 139 – 147.

Tips
- Encourage the children to watch your mouth for placement cues.

- Form the alphabet sign near your face to keep the children's attention focused on your face.

- Repeat the sound distinctly three times with a short pause between the repetitions. Prolong continuant sounds, repeating each prolongation three times.

- Present the long vowel sound first, then the short vowel sound.

- The letter C makes the /k/ and the /s/ sound. Present both sounds.

- Present both the voiced and voiceless /th/ sounds.

- Develop a definite cadence to your alphabet review to provide prosodic support.

- Refer to a graphic representation of each letter (e.g., point to the letter on an alphabet chart, place a magnetic letter on a board, use an alphabet puzzle, write the letter on a chalkboard).

❹ Drill Multisyllabic Words

Drill is the most important factor for success in improving the intelligibility of children with apraxia. The children will come to expect drill as part of the program. Don't let them talk you out of it.

Practice the ABC Flash Cards at the Multisyllabic Words level. Include practice of the challenging context when the target is easily produced. Record the accuracy of each child's response (+/–) on the Apraxia Group Response Form, page 151, or the Apraxia Individual Response Form, page 153. Use the Supplemental Target List on page 81 for alternative words or for additional practice.

Tips
- Encourage correct articulation of all sounds in the multisyllabic word.

- Establish a rapid pace.

- Elicit a high number of responses.

- Require three to five unison responses, followed by an individual response from each child.

- Cue the initial sound of each syllable using the alphabet signs.

- Do not dwell on difficult words. Provide a model and production cues and then go on.

- Elicit the target word in a more complex context (the suggested carrier phrase).

- If necessary, use a simple, quick, tangible reinforcer to keep the children on task. (See page 149.)

❺ Words of Increasing Length

Ask the children to repeat the following syllable groups until the whole utterance has been produced, cueing difficult sounds with the alphabet signs. Use hand gestures to establish an echoing routine. After practicing the whole utterance a few times, call on an individual child to use the utterance in response to the role play. Encourage dynamic expression.

- E - EI - EIE - EIEI - EIEIO!

  Role Play: Alejandro, finish the song: "Old MacDonald had a farm . . . ."

- ya - yaba - yabada - yabadaba - yabadabadoo!

  Role Play: Dante, what does Fred Flintstone say?

- ab - abbra - abbraca - abbracada - abbracadabra!

  Role Play: Erin, the magician pulls a rabbit out of his hat. What does he say?

- I'm - I'm go - I'm gonna - I'm gonna get - I'm gonna get you!

  Role Play: Becca, Daddy likes to play a tickle game with you. What does he say?

- Row - Row, row - Row, row, row - Row, row, row your - Row, row, row your boat.

  Role Play: Hayley, everyone knows this song. Can you sing it?

❻ Song

Sing a familiar song with the children that repeats a multisyllabic word. Sing the song slowly with accentuated rhythm. Cue difficult sounds in key words with the alphabet signs. A rhythmic, whole-body movement, such as swinging or clapping to the beat of the song, will facilitate word production. Song suggestions include:

Teddy Bear, Teddy Bear

"Teddy Bear, Teddy Bear, turn around.
Teddy Bear, Teddy Bear, touch the ground.
Teddy Bear, Teddy Bear, shine my shoe.
Teddy Bear, Teddy Bear, that will do."

Hickory, Dickory, Dock

"Hickory, dickory, dock.
The mouse ran up the clock.
The clock struck one.
The mouse ran down.
Hickory, dickory, dock."

John Jacob Jingleheimer Schmidt

"John Jacob Jingleheimer Schmidt,
His name is my name too.
Whenever we go out
The people always shout,
'John Jacob Jingleheimer Schmidt.'
Dah dah dah dah dah dah dah."

❼ Closure

Invite the parents/caregivers into the therapy room. Discuss the session and distribute the ABC Flash Cards, pages 73 – 80, Family Letter, page 82, Home Practice Log, page 83, and Home Practice Notes, page 84. Stress the importance of daily practice and remind the parents/caregivers to complete the home practice logs and notes. Suggest that the family sing the song used in therapy and read the books listed on the letter for additional practice and carryover. The songs and books should be presented slowly and with exaggerated rhythm and expression so the children have an opportunity to join in. Once the child is familiar with the song or book, the parent/caregiver should pause frequently to allow the child to fill in the multisyllabic word.

On the last day of the phase, present a Phase Completion Certificate to each child, page 85.

Oral Motor Exercises — Mouth Postures

Lip Exercises

Kiss the palm of your hand. Then blow a kiss.

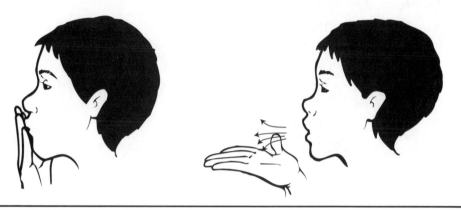

Make slow lip pops, then fast ones.

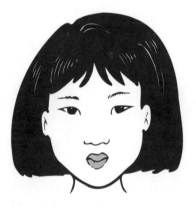

Hide your upper lip with your lower lip. Then hide your lower lip with your upper lip.

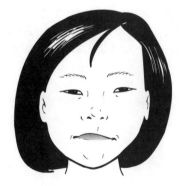 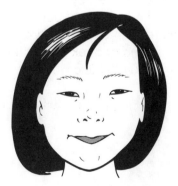

Oral Motor Exercises — Mouth Postures, continued

Tongue Exercises

Point your tongue toward your chin. Then move it toward your nose. Try to stretch your tongue a little farther each time.

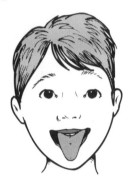 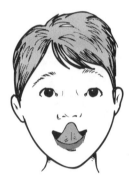

Use your tongue tip to circle your lips. Go in one direction and then the other. Don't miss the corners of your lips.

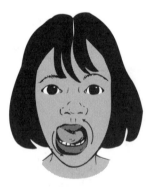 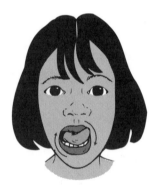

Curl up the sides of your tongue. Then move your tongue in and out of your mouth.

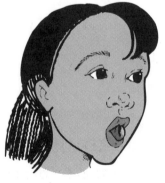 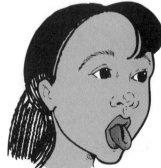

ABC Flash Cards

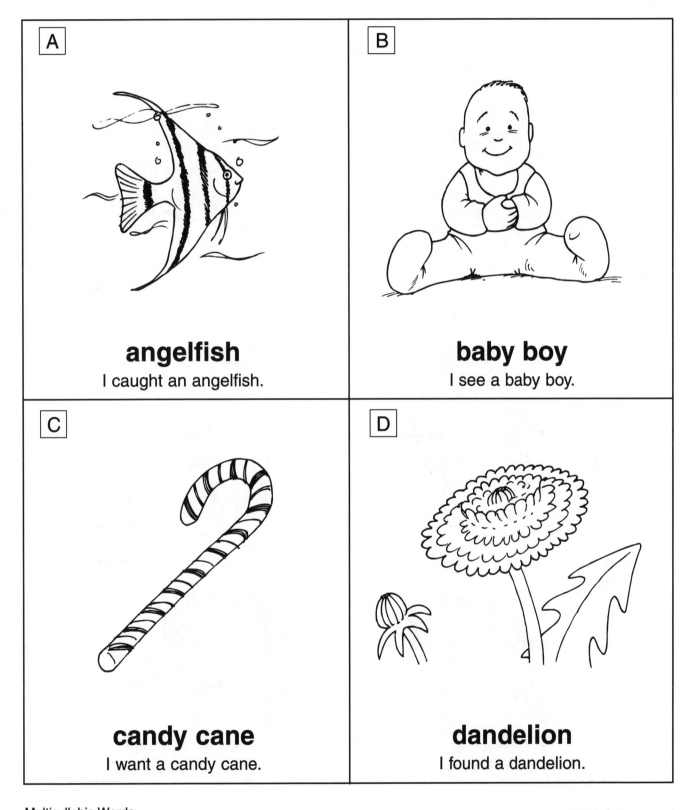

A

angelfish
I caught an angelfish.

B

baby boy
I see a baby boy.

C

candy cane
I want a candy cane.

D

dandelion
I found a dandelion.

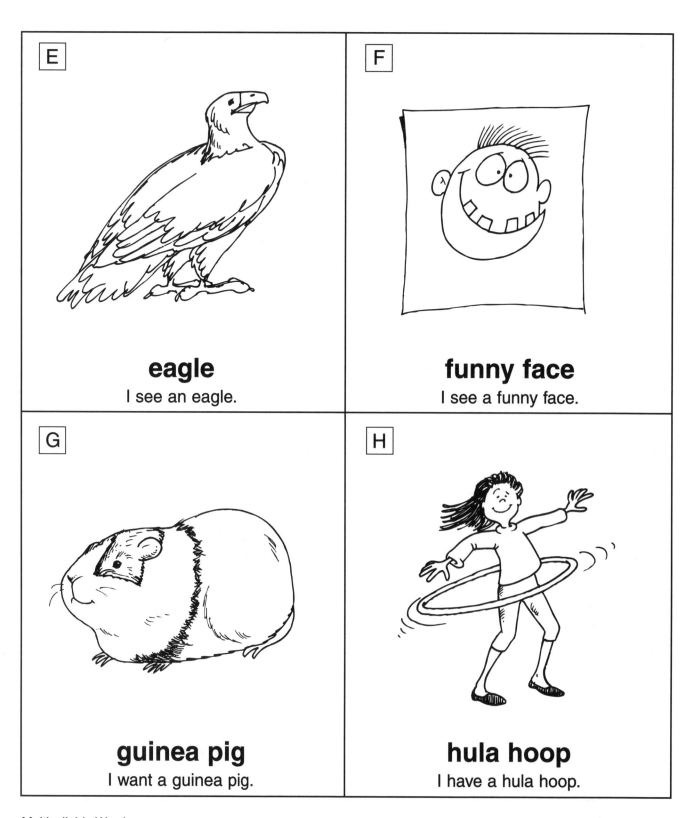

E

eagle
I see an eagle.

F

funny face
I see a funny face.

G

guinea pig
I want a guinea pig.

H

hula hoop
I have a hula hoop.

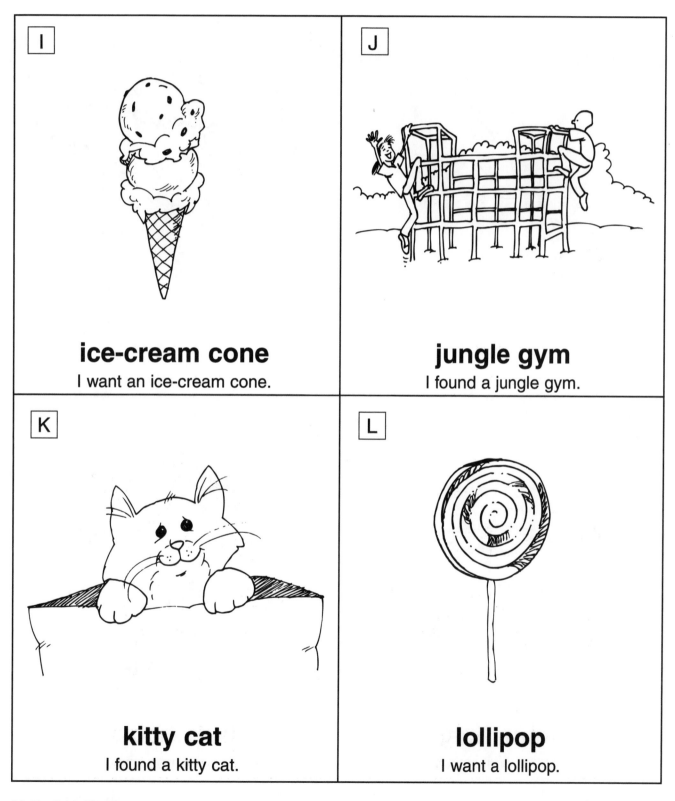

ice-cream cone
I want an ice-cream cone.

jungle gym
I found a jungle gym.

kitty cat
I found a kitty cat.

lollipop
I want a lollipop.

Multisyllabic Words
Just for Kids: Apraxia   75

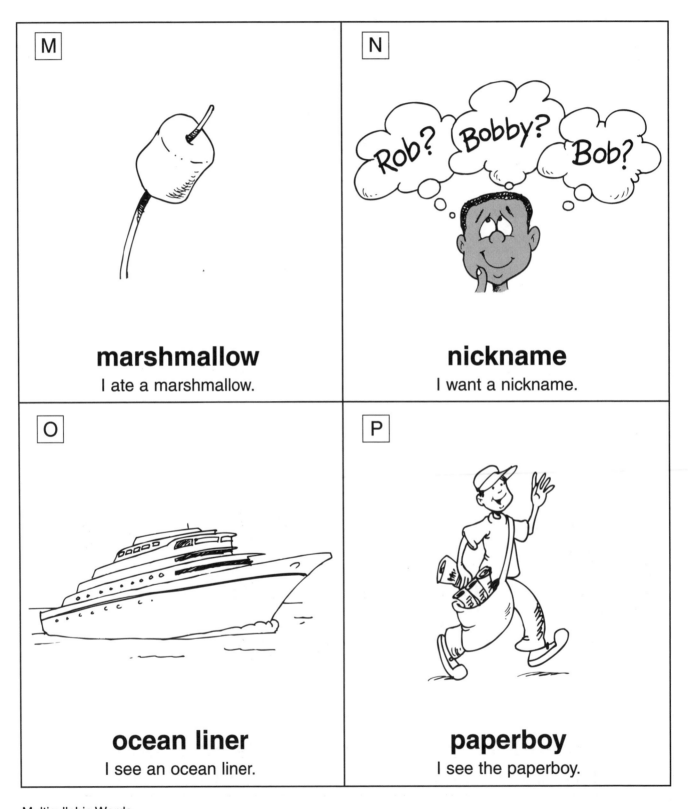

M

marshmallow

I ate a marshmallow.

N

nickname

I want a nickname.

O

ocean liner

I see an ocean liner.

P

paperboy

I see the paperboy.

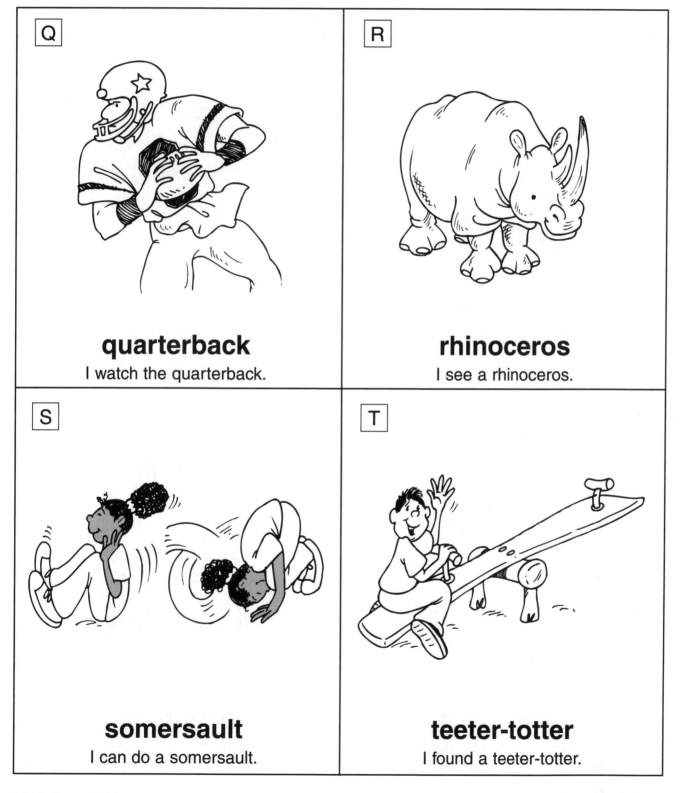

Q

quarterback

I watch the quarterback.

R

rhinoceros

I see a rhinoceros.

S

somersault

I can do a somersault.

T

teeter-totter

I found a teeter-totter.

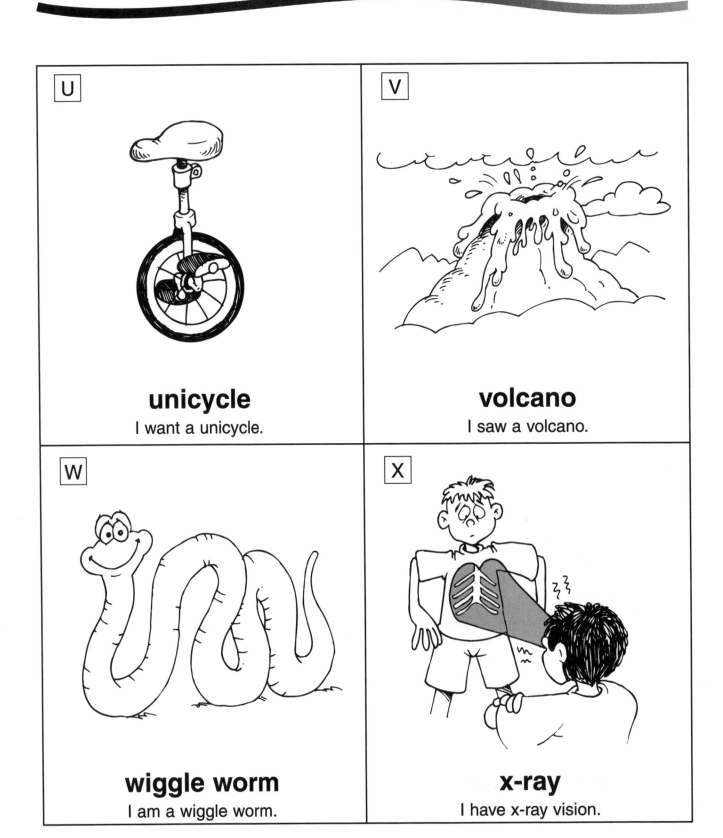

U

unicycle

I want a unicycle.

V

volcano

I saw a volcano.

W

wiggle worm

I am a wiggle worm.

X

x-ray

I have x-ray vision.

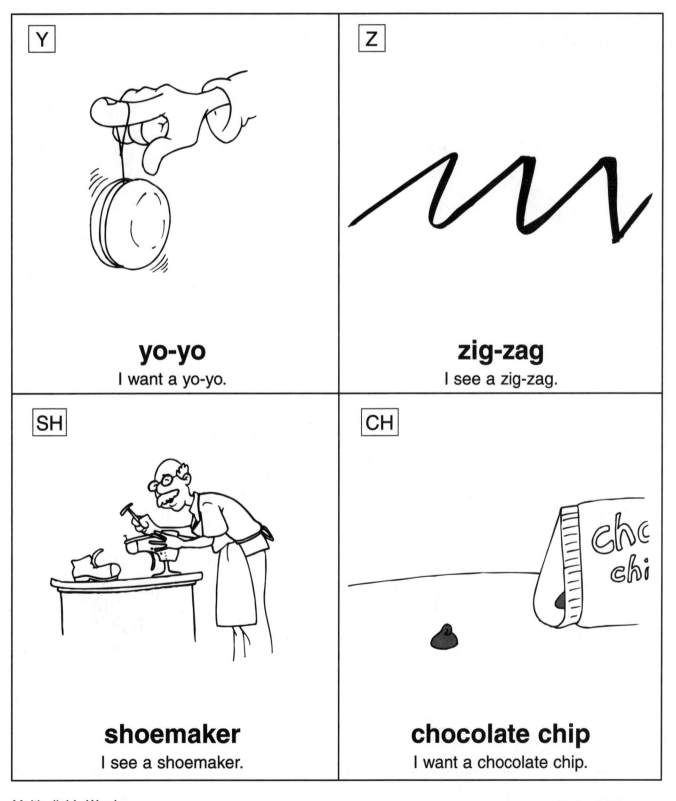

Y

yo-yo
I want a yo-yo.

Z

zig-zag
I see a zig-zag.

SH

shoemaker
I see a shoemaker.

CH

chocolate chip
I want a chocolate chip.

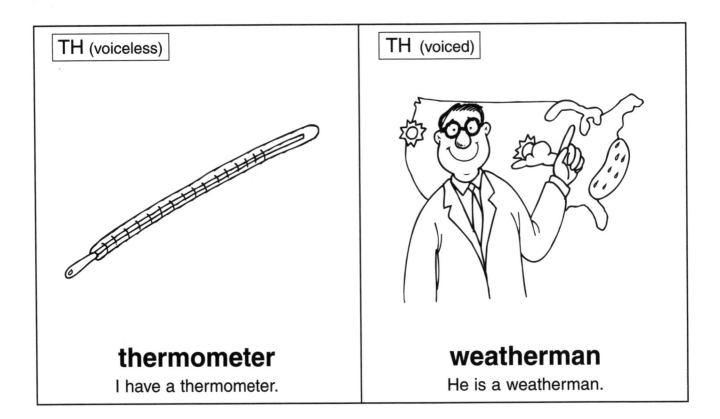

TH (voiceless)

TH (voiced)

thermometer

I have a thermometer.

weatherman

He is a weatherman.

Supplemental Target List

Use these words as alternatives for the multisyllabic words on the ABC Flash Cards or for additional practice.

A — airplane, airport

B — bumblebee, butterfly, basketball, banana, bicycle, bowling ball

C — candy bar, calendar, cantaloupe, cucumber, cocoa, cookie cutter

D — dinosaur, dynamite, dangerous, December, donut

E — eagle, evening, Egypt, easy

F — fireplace, firefly, fingernail, footprint

G — garden, gumdrop, gasoline, gorilla

H — helicopter, hummingbird, honeybee, hamburger, hurricane

I — eyelash, eyeball, icicle, idea

J — janitor, jellyfish, Japanese, gentleman, jewelry

K — kitchen sink, kindergarten, kangaroo, Kentucky

L — ladybug, lawn mower, lima bean, lemonade

M — medicine, music box, marshmallow, Mickey Mouse®

N — nobody, November, napkin holder, newspaper, neighborhood

O — okay, Olympics, oak tree, ozone layer

P — piano, pajamas, peppermint, paperboy, peanut butter, porcupine

Q — quiet, question mark, quarter

R — radio, rectangle, Robin Hood, rattlesnake, rodeo

S — soccer ball, Saturday, Superman, safety pin, souvenir

T — television, tornado, tambourine, telephone, tangerine

U — unicorn, uniform, unison, university

W — watermelon, wigwam, winter hat, World Wide Web, woodwork

X — excellent, exercise, exit, extraordinary

Y — yo-yo, yard line, yesterday, Yellowstone, Yogi Bear®

Z — zookeeper, xylophone, zebra fish, zucchini

SH — shampoo, shopping bag, shipshape, shower cap, shivering

CH — choo-choo train, cheddar cheese, chimney, chapter book

voiceless TH — thingamagig, thunderstorm, thumbnail, thundershower

voiced TH — grandmother, grandfather, brother

Dear Family,

Today we began Phase Three of your child's speech therapy program. It is called Multisyllabic Words. Your child is learning to connect the sounds and syllables in two- to four-syllable words.

I am once again sending home flash cards and home practice materials. Please practice the flash cards every day with your child. You can help your child by clapping out the syllables as you say the word, finding the little word within the big word, like *mom* in *thermometer*, and by stressing the accented syllable. It will also be helpful to form the alphabet sign for the first letter of each syllable. Don't become discouraged if this phase is particularly difficult for your child. Practice truly does make perfect! Once your child can say the multisyllabic word easily, try the phrase included on the flashcard. Remember to complete the Home Practice Log and a Home Practice Note every time you drill the ABC Flash Cards with your child.

Besides drilling the flash cards, you can practice multisyllabic words in other ways. You can sing songs and read books that contain many two- to four-syllable words. Here are a few suggestions:

Songs
- *Teddy Bear, Teddy Bear*
- *Hickory Dickory Dock*
- *John Jacob Jingleheimer Schmidt*

Books
- *The Lady with the Alligator Purse* adapted and illustrated by Nadine Bernard Westcott
- *Peanut Butter and Jelly: A Play Rhyme* illustrated by Nadine Bernard Westcott
- *The Very Hungry Caterpillar* by Eric Carle
- *Polar Bear, Polar Bear, What Do You Hear?* by Bill Martin Jr and Eric Carle

Thank you for your support. Please call if you have questions or concerns. You are always welcome to observe your child in therapy.

Sincerely,

_____

Speech-Language Pathologist

_____

Phone

Home Practice Log

Child: _____ Speech-Language Pathologist: _____

Parent/Caregiver: Please practice the ABC Flash Cards at the Multisyllabic Words level with your child daily (at least 5 days per week). Mark a **+** in the box when your child pronounces the multi-syllabic word correctly; mark a **–** in the box when your child incorrectly pronounces the multisyllabic word. Record the total number of correct responses in the box at the bottom of the column. Please return this log when completed or at the end of this phase. Thanks!

Date															
A															
B															
C															
D															
E															
F															
G															
H															
I															
J															
K															
L															
M															
N															
O															
P															
Q															
R															
S															
T															
U															
V															
W															
X															
Y															
Z															
SH															
CH															
TH (voiceless)															
TH (voiced)															
Total Correct															

Multisyllabic Words
Just for Kids: Apraxia

83

Home Practice Notes

Parent/Caregiver: Please complete a Home Practice Note after each practice session with your child. Record the number of correct responses from the Home Practice Log in the space provided. Ask your child to return the note to speech therapy for a reward. Thanks!

We practiced the ABC Flash Cards at the Multisyllabic Words level today.

_____ pronounced _____ words correctly!
Child   *number*

_____   _____
Parent/Caregiver Signature   *Date*

(Please return to Speech-Language Therapy.)   ☐ Send more notes.

We practiced the ABC Flash Cards at the Multisyllabic Words level today.

_____ pronounced _____ words correctly!
Child   *number*

_____   _____
Parent/Caregiver Signature   *Date*

(Please return to Speech-Language Therapy.)   ☐ Send more notes.

We practiced the ABC Flash Cards at the Multisyllabic Words level today.

_____ pronounced _____ words correctly!
Child   *number*

_____   _____
Parent/Caregiver Signature   *Date*

(Please return to Speech-Language Therapy.)   ☐ Send more notes.

We practiced the ABC Flash Cards at the Multisyllabic Words level today.

_____ pronounced _____ words correctly!
Child   *number*

_____   _____
Parent/Caregiver Signature   *Date*

(Please return to Speech-Language Therapy.)   ☐ Send more notes.

We practiced the ABC Flash Cards at the Multisyllabic Words level today.

_____ pronounced _____ words correctly!
Child   *number*

_____   _____
Parent/Caregiver Signature   *Date*

(Please return to Speech-Language Therapy.)   ☐ Send more notes.

---

dandelion • bumble bee • chocolate chip • lollipop

Multisyllabic Words

This is to certify that

_____

has successfully completed

Phase Three of the

Apraxia Therapy Program.

_____
Speech-Language Pathologist

_____
Date

• dandelion • bumble bee • lollipop

• dandelion • bumble bee • chocolate chip • lollipop

lollipop • dandelion • chocolate chip •

Phase Completion Certificate
Just for Kids: Apraxia

Sentences
Phase Four

Rationale

Sentences: Phase Four increases the syntactic and linguistic load of the utterance. Sound sequences are stressed in Phase Four along with grammar, syntax, and vocabulary. Children with apraxia of speech often display poor syntactical and linguistic development. They seem to let their syntax and vocabulary go because it requires too much effort to make themselves understood. Their speech often consists of short phrases, limited stereotypic sentence types, and immature vocabulary.

At this point in the program, the children should be handling movement transitions in words and short phrases more successfully. Now they need to attend to the grammatical and syntactical components of speech. Do not simplify the sentences by making errors in grammar and syntax. It is important to look at the whole child as a communicator. At the end of the program, you do not want the children's speech to be filled with grammatical and syntactical errors. To increase demands on the children for easily-produced sentences, ask them to repeat the sentence after an imposed delay (i.e., the question included on the flash card). The delay will require them to remember the phonetic, syntactic, and linguistic elements of the sentence.

Strategies

Attending to phonetic, syntactic, and linguistic aspects of sentences will be challenging for the children. The following strategies will be helpful.

- Use the alphabet signs to cue difficult sounds.

- Make cards with three, four, five, and six stickers on them. Draw attention to individual words within the sentence by touching a sticker on the appropriate card for each word.

- Highlight difficult words by adding stress. For example, "**She** is happy."

- Repeat a difficult grammatical form in a variety of sentences until the children achieve success.

  For example:
  "Michelle is wearing a red dress."
  "Michelle is eating an apple."
  "Michelle is playing the piano."

- Provide positive specific feedback. For example, "All of your sounds were right. Now let's try to include the word *is*."

- Give the children adequate time to formulate and self-correct their responses.

Criterion for Moving to Phase Five

The complete sentence must be correct in Phase Four to score it correct, including the sounds, grammar, word order, and vocabulary. A 75-80% proficiency level should be achieved before moving to Phase Five of the program. If a particular child has more difficulty than others with grammar, you may simplify the sentence, but do not break grammar rules to do so.

Instructional Tools

Oral-Motor Mouth Postures

Pictures of lip and tongue placement for the oral-motor exercises in Phase Four are provided on pages 93 – 94. Use the pictures for additional visual support when doing the exercises.

ABC Flash Cards

The flash cards in Phase Four show a sentence, a picture, and a question. The sentence is the target; the question is asked as an imposed delay for the challenging context. (See pages 95 – 102.)

Supplemental Target List

A supplemental list of sentences is provided on pages 103 – 105. Use this list for alternative sentences or additional practice.

Family Letter and Home Practice Materials

The Family Letter, page 106, briefly describes Phase Four and suggests ways for the parents/ caregivers to work with their child at home. Attach a copy of the ABC Flash Cards at the Sentences level, pages 95 – 102, the Home Practice Log, page 107, and Home Practice Notes, page 108. Send these materials home with the children after the first session of the phase.

Phase Completion Certificate

Present the certificate, page 109, to the children when they complete Phase Four.

Phase Four Therapy

Materials
- Alphabet Mouth Postures, pages 139 – 147
- laminated set of ABC Flash Cards, pages 95 – 102, for use in therapy
- Oral-Motor Exercises – Mouth Postures, pages 93 – 94
- small, hand-held mirror for each child
- reinforcement activity, if needed, page 149
- Apraxia Group Response Form, page 151, or Apraxia Individual Response Form, page 153
- one set of ABC Flash Cards for each child, pages 95 – 102, for practice at home
- one Family Letter, Home Practice Log, and Home Practice Notes for each child, pages 106 – 108
- Phase Completion Certificate for each child, page 109
- Supplemental Target List, pages 103 – 105 (optional)

Session Sequence

❶ Gross Motor Warm-Up

Ask the children to perform a gross motor movement such as running in place, clapping, or doing jumping jacks while singing the ABC song. (See page 148 for additional gross motor movement activities.) Sing the song slowly with exaggerated articulation. Repeat the song and movement activity several times.

> "A, B, C, D, E, F, G,
> H, I, J, K, L-M-N-O-P,
> Q, R, S,
> T, U, V,
> W, X, Y, and Z.
> Now I know my ABCs.
> Next time won't you sing with me?"

❷ Oral-Motor Exercises

Ask the children to imitate the following lip and tongue exercises five times each. Display the mouth posture pictures on pages 93 – 94. Encourage the children to match the postures as they perform the exercises. Children may benefit from using their mirrors. Use your fingers to indicate the number of repetitions.

Lip Exercises
- Puff out your cheeks with air. Hold your lips tight to keep the air in.

- Give a long, squeaky kiss.

- Raise and stretch your upper lip to show your top teeth. Then lower and stretch your lower lip to show your bottom teeth.

Tongue Exercises

- Rub the "spot" (alveolar ridge) with your finger. Then rub it with the tip of your tongue.

- Rub the "pocket" (the area behind your bottom teeth) with your finger. Then rub it with the tip of your tongue.

- Touch the tip of your tongue to the "pocket." Then touch it to the "spot."

❸ Alphabet Chant

Recite the alphabet in unison with the children using the Alphabet Chant found on pages 137 – 138. The chant requires the children to form the sign, say the letter name, and produce the associated sound(s). Use hand-over-hand assistance, if necessary, to form the signs. Show the Alphabet Mouth Posture pictures for added visual support in producing the sounds, pages 139 – 147.

Tips
- Encourage the children to watch your mouth for placement cues.

- Form the alphabet sign near your face to keep the children's attention focused on your face.

- Repeat the sound distinctly three times with a short pause between the repetitions. Prolong continuant sounds, repeating each prolongation three times.

- Present the long vowel sound first, then the short vowel sound.

- The letter C makes the /k/ and the /s/ sound. Present both sounds.

- Present both the voiced and voiceless /th/ sounds.

- Develop a definite cadence to your alphabet review to provide prosodic support.

- Refer to a graphic representation of each letter (e.g., point to the letter on an alphabet chart, place a magnetic letter on a board, use an alphabet puzzle, write the letter on a chalkboard).

❹ Drill Sentences

Drill is the most important factor for success in improving the intelligibility of children with apraxia. The children will come to expect drill as part of the program. Don't let them talk you out of it.

Practice the ABC Flash Cards at the Sentences level. Include practice of the challenging context when the target is easily produced. Record the accuracy of each child's response (+/–) on the Apraxia Group Response Form, page 151, or the Apraxia Individual Response Form, page 153. Use the Supplemental Target List on pages 103 – 105 for alternative sentences or for additional practice.

Tips   • Encourage correct articulation of all sounds in the sentence.

• Establish a rapid pace of stimulus presentation.

• Elicit a high number of responses.

• Require three to five unison responses, followed by an individual response from each child.

• Cue difficult sounds using the alphabet signs.

• Do not dwell on difficult sentences. Provide a model and production cues, then go on.

• If necessary, simplify difficult sentences, but do not make errors in grammar and syntax.

• If necessary, use a simple, quick, tangible reinforcer to keep the children on task. (See page 149.)

5 Words of Increasing Length

Ask the children to repeat the following syllable groups until the whole utterance has been produced, cueing difficult sounds with the alphabet signs. Use hand gestures to establish an echoing routine. After practicing the whole utterance a few times, call on an individual child to use the utterance in response to the role play. Encourage dynamic expression.

• Een - Eensy - Eensy-ween - Eensy-weensy - Eensy-weensy spi - Eensy-weensy spider!

    Role Play: Johnna, what climbs up the waterspout? The . . . .

• Tra - Tra la - Tra la la - Tra la la boom - Tra la la boom dee - Tra la la boom dee ay!

    Role Play: Stevie, the circus is coming to town. What song will the clowns sing?

• Sing - Sing a - Sing a song - Sing a song of - Sing a song of six - Sing a song of sixpence!

    Role Play: Cameron, I know a song about blackbirds. Can you start it?

• Hap - Happy - Happy birth - Happy birthday - Happy birthday to - Happy birthday to you!

    Role Play: Chaz, it's my birthday. What do you say to me?

• O - Okey - Okey do - Okey dokey - Okey dokey, Smo - Okey dokey, Smokey!

    Role Play: Devon, let's go swimming. What do you say?

❻ Song

Sing a familiar song with the children that repeats a phrase or sentence several times in its chorus. Sing the song slowly with accentuated rhythm. Cue difficult sounds in key words with the alphabet signs. A rhythmic, whole-body movement, such as swinging or clapping to the beat of the song, will facilitate phrase and sentence production. Song suggestions include:

Row, Row, Row Your Boat

"Row, row, row your boat,
Gently down the stream.
Merrily, merrily, merrily, merrily,
Life is but a dream."

The Farmer in the Dell

"The farmer in the dell,
The farmer in the dell,
Heigh-ho the derry-O!
The farmer in the dell.

"The farmer takes a wife.
The farmer takes a wife.
Heigh-ho the derry-O!
The farmer takes a wife.

"The wife takes the child.
The wife takes the child.
Heigh-ho the derry-O!
The wife takes the child.

"The child takes the nurse.
The child takes the nurse.
Heigh-ho the derry-O!
The child takes the nurse.

"The nurse takes the dog.
The nurse takes the dog.
Heigh-ho the derry-O!
The nurse takes the dog.

"The dog takes the cat.
The dog takes the cat.
Heigh-ho the derry-O!
The dog takes the cat.

"The cat takes the rat.
The cat takes the rat.
Heigh-ho the derry-O!
The cat takes the rat.

"The rat takes the cheese.
The rat takes the cheese.
Heigh-ho the derry-O!
The rat takes the cheese.

"The cheese stands alone.
The cheese stands alone.
Heigh-ho the derry-O!
The cheese stands alone."

The Mulberry Bush

"Here we go 'round the mulberry bush, the mulberry bush, the mulberry bush.
Here we go 'round the mulberry bush, so early in the morning.

"This is the way we wash our clothes, wash our clothes, wash our clothes.
This is the way we wash our clothes, so early in the morning.

"This is the way we iron our clothes, iron our clothes, iron our clothes.
This is the way we iron our clothes, so early in the morning.

"This is the way we scrub the floor, scrub the floor, scrub the floor.
This is the way we scrub the floor, so early in the morning.

"This is the way we mend our clothes, mend our clothes, mend our clothes.
This is the way we mend our clothes, so early in the morning.

"This is the way we sweep the house, sweep the house, sweep the house.
This is the way we sweep the house, so early in the morning.

"This is the way we bake our bread, bake our bread, bake our bread.
This is the way we bake our bread, so early in the morning.

"This is the way we read a book, read a book, read a book.
This is the way we read a book, so early in the morning."

❼ Closure

Invite the parents/caregivers into the therapy room. Discuss the session and distribute the ABC Flash Cards, pages 95 – 102, Family Letter, page 106, Home Practice Log, page 107, and Home Practice Notes, page 108. Stress the importance of daily practice and remind the parents/caregivers to complete the home practice logs and notes. Suggest that the family sing the song used in therapy and read the books listed on the letter for additional practice and carryover. The songs and books should be presented slowly and with exaggerated rhythm and expression so the children have an opportunity to join in. Once the child is familiar with the song or book, the parent/caregiver should pause frequently to allow the child to fill in the repetitive phrases/sentences.

On the last day of the phase, present a Phase Completion Certificate to each child, page 109.

Oral Motor Exercises — Mouth Postures

Lip Exercises

Puff out your cheeks with air. Hold your lips tight to keep the air in.

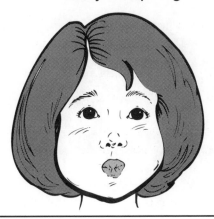

Give a long, squeaky kiss.

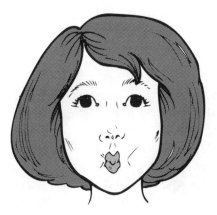

Raise and stretch your upper lip to show your top teeth. Then lower and stretch your lower lip to show your bottom teeth.

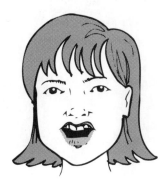 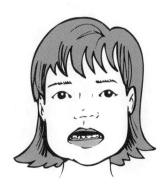

Tongue Exercises

Rub the "spot" (alveolar ridge) with your finger. Then rub it with the tip of your tongue.

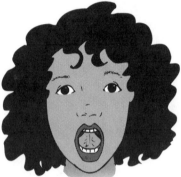

Rub the "pocket" (the area behind your bottom teeth) with your finger. Then rub it with the tip of your tongue.

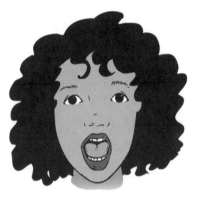

Touch the tip of your tongue to the "pocket." Then touch it to the "spot."

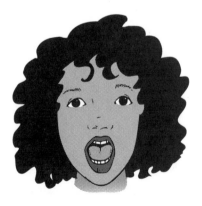
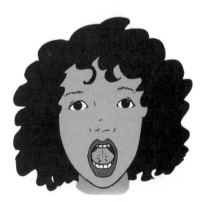

ABC Flash Cards

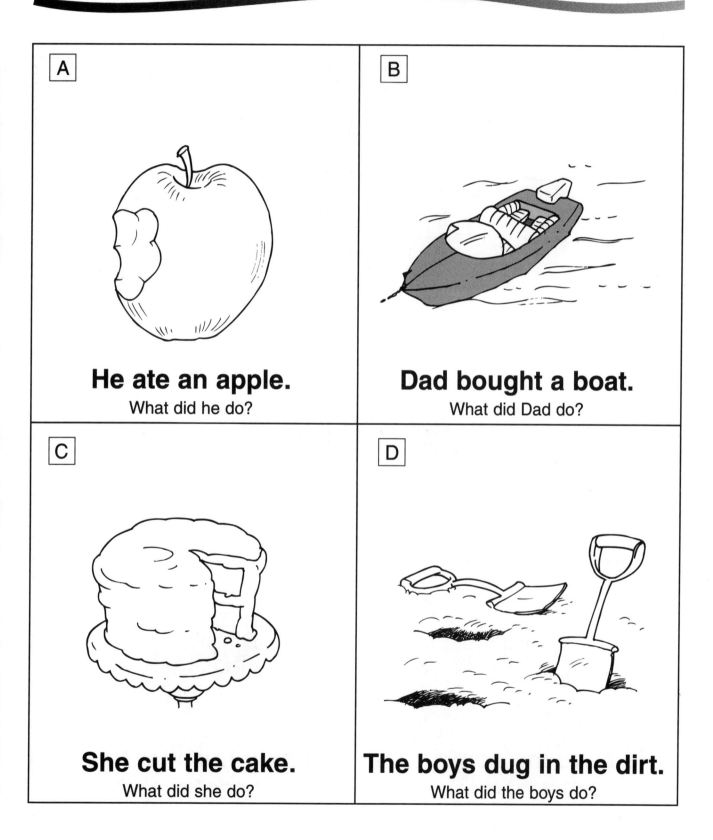

A

He ate an apple.
What did he do?

B

Dad bought a boat.
What did Dad do?

C

She cut the cake.
What did she do?

D

The boys dug in the dirt.
What did the boys do?

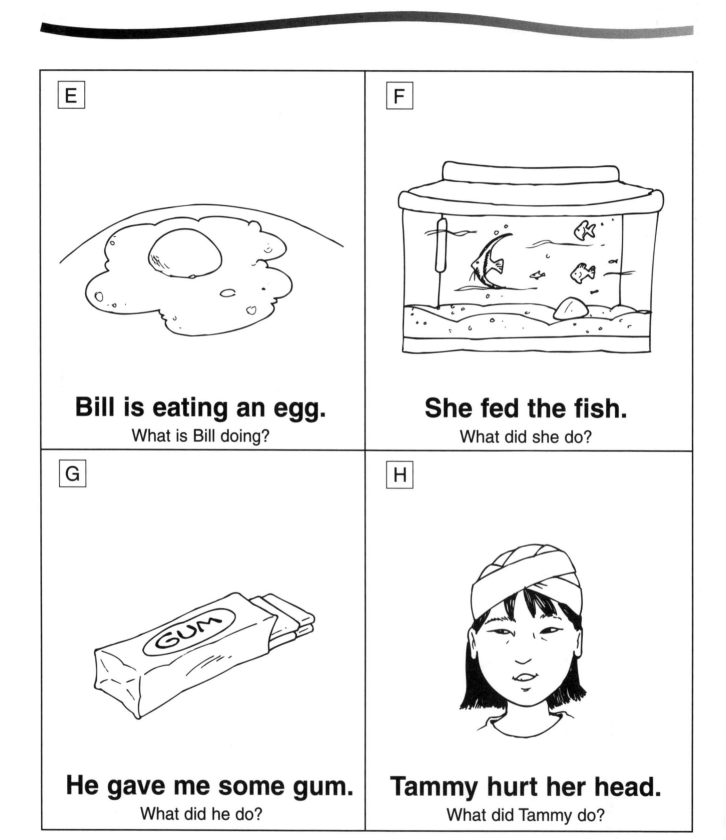

E

Bill is eating an egg.

What is Bill doing?

F

She fed the fish.

What did she do?

G

He gave me some gum.

What did he do?

H

Tammy hurt her head.

What did Tammy do?

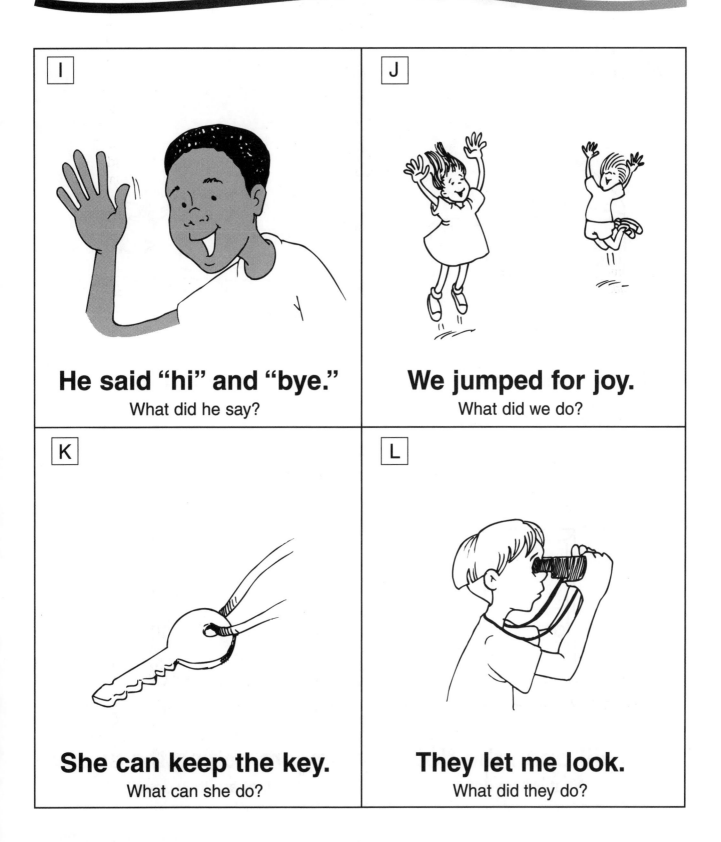

I

He said "hi" and "bye."

What did he say?

J

We jumped for joy.

What did we do?

K

She can keep the key.

What can she do?

L

They let me look.

What did they do?

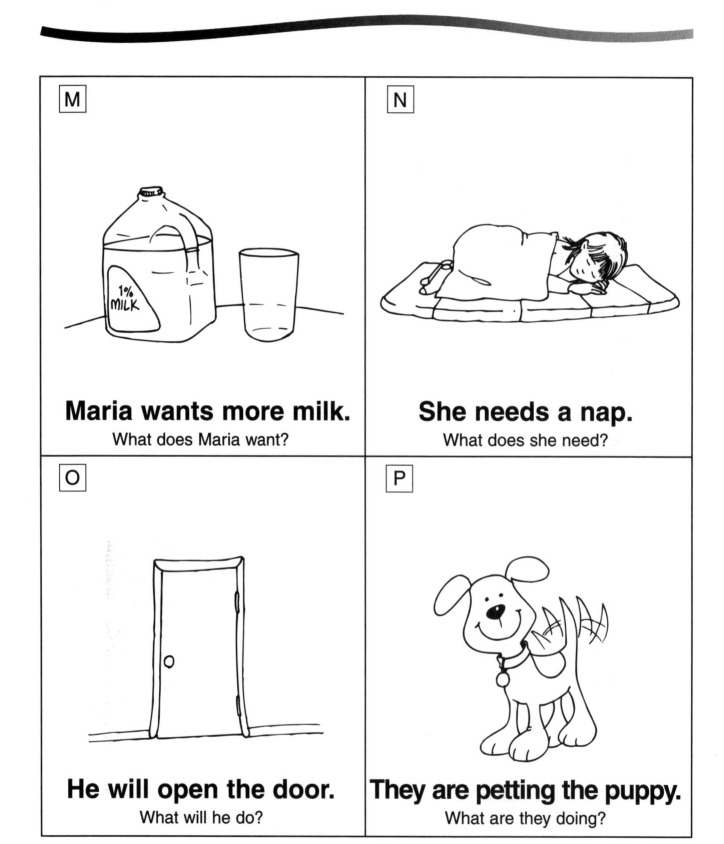

M

Maria wants more milk.
What does Maria want?

N

She needs a nap.
What does she need?

O

He will open the door.
What will he do?

P

They are petting the puppy.
What are they doing?

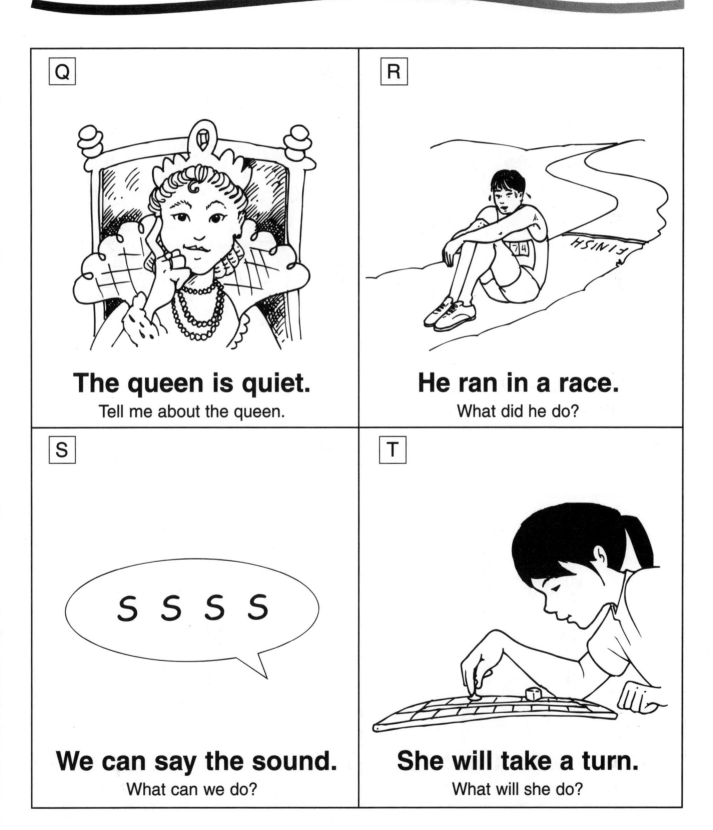

Q

The queen is quiet.
Tell me about the queen.

R

He ran in a race.
What did he do?

S

S S S S

We can say the sound.
What can we do?

T

She will take a turn.
What will she do?

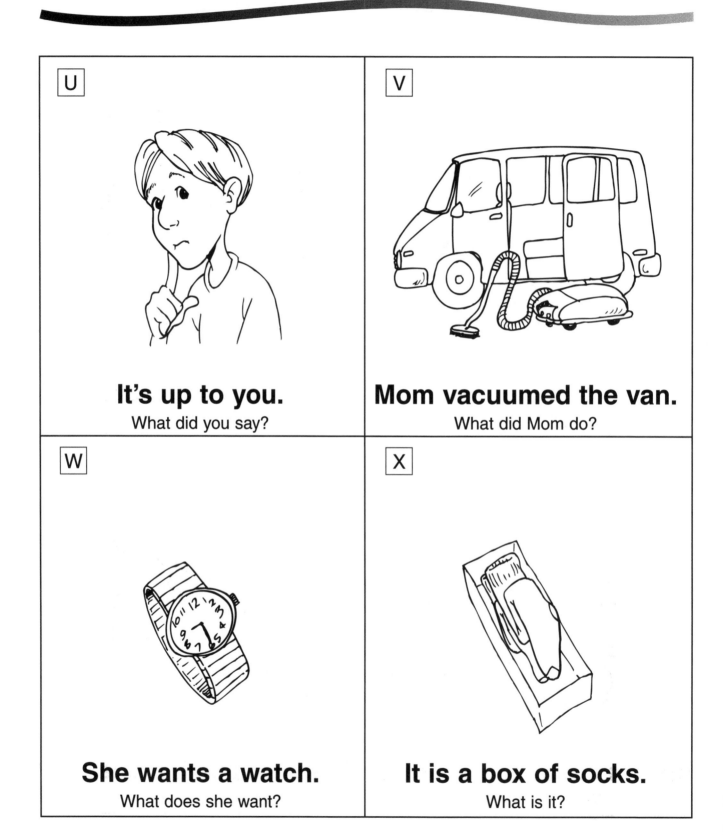

U

It's up to you.
What did you say?

V

Mom vacuumed the van.
What did Mom do?

W

She wants a watch.
What does she want?

X

It is a box of socks.
What is it?

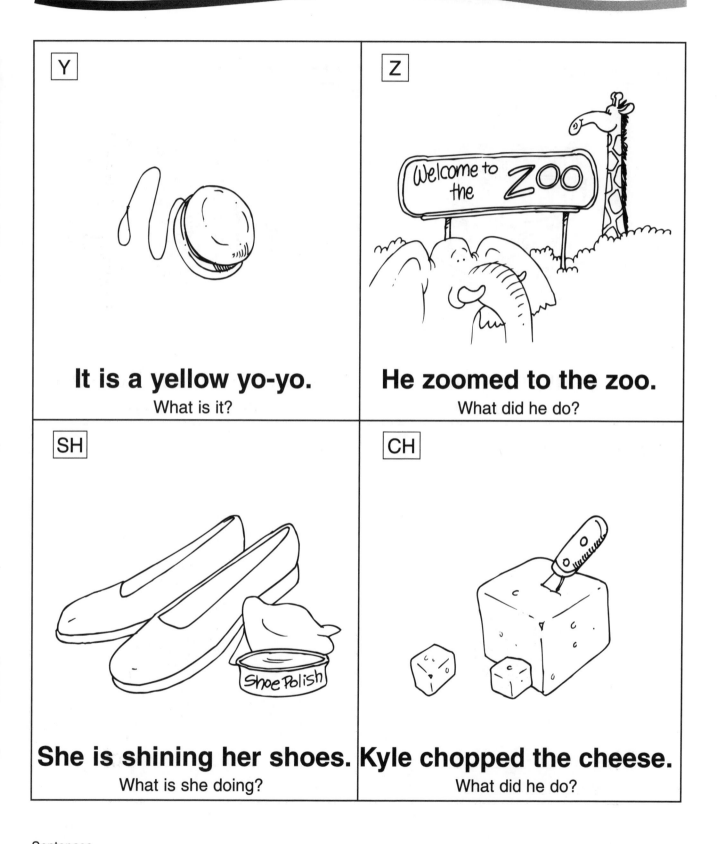

Y

It is a yellow yo-yo.

What is it?

Z

He zoomed to the zoo.

What did he do?

SH

She is shining her shoes.

What is she doing?

CH

Kyle chopped the cheese.

What did he do?

TH (voiceless)

Is it thick or thin?
What did you ask?

TH (voiced)

Give them their tickets.
What should I give them?

Supplemental Target List

Use these sentences as alternatives for the sentences on the ABC Flash Cards or for additional practice.

A — He acted like an ape.
   Her arm ached.
   You are an angel.

B — I saw a baby bear.
   He needs a bat and ball.
   She brought a book to the beach.

C — He is coming to camp.
   I am counting the cows.
   We kept the cat.

D — She dusted the desk.
   He is dozing on the deck.
   The dog dashed away.

E — Ed cut his ear.
   It was easy in the end.
   The eagle sat on the edge.

F — They had fun at the fair.
   He found a fan.
   She feels fine.

G — She gave me a gift.
   He is getting gas.
   They had a good game.

H — I will hike up the hill.
   He helped his mom.
   She is holding her hat.

I — I bought some ice.
   It is a good idea.
   I am rubbing my eyes.

J — Jake rode on a jet.
   She told a joke at her job.
   I broke the jelly jar.

K — He kicked the can.
     I kissed my cousin.
     Can you make a kite?

L — She likes the lake.
     They looked at their lawn.
     He has a loud laugh.

M —He made me mad.
     We missed the movie.
     The mittens are mine.

N — The nurse is nice.
     She heard a noise at night.
     He knows my name.

O — I did it on my own.
     Is four even or odd?
     The dog obeys his owner.

P — Can you peel the peach?
     I put it in your purse.
     He will pay for the pop.

Q — It was a quick quiz.
     He quit asking questions.
     A duck says, "quack-quack."

R — I am reading a recipe.
     They are renting a red house.
     I can't reach the reins.

S — He sipped his soup.
     She sees a seal.
     I will save a seat.

T — She told a tall tale.
     They are going to town.
     It's on the tip of my tongue.

U — You look unhappy.
     My uncle is visiting us.
     They sat under the umbrella.

V — He voted for Vic.
Is the vent open?
Vera has a good voice.

W — I walked through the weeds.
She woke up weak.
He will win the race.

X — He locks the box.
Can you fix the mixer?
We found the exit.

Y — Are you done yet?
The yogurt tastes yummy.
I used to like yams.

Z — I zipped my zipper.
It zigged and zagged.
The zebra lives at the zoo.

SH — She is going shopping.
He is shearing the sheep.
We should go to a show.

CH — The dog is chasing the chipmunk.
Chuck checked his math.
The child's cheeks are red.

TH (voiceless) — I think he's a thief.
Thad said, "Thanks."
I thought you were thirsty.

TH (voiced) — They did it by themselves.
They should stop that.
Put those shoes there.

Dear Family,

Today we began Phase Four of your child's speech therapy program. Your child is learning to use correct grammar as well as sounds in sentences. Children with apraxia often let their grammar go because all their energy goes into trying to make themselves understood.

I am sending home flash cards with sentences written on them and home practice materials. Please practice the flash cards every day with your child. Review each sentence several times until your child can say it with the correct sounds and grammar. For sentences your child can produce easily, also ask the question included on the card. It will require your child to remember the sound sequences and grammar after a short delay. Continue to complete the Home Practice Log and a Home Practice Note every time you drill the ABC Flash Cards with your child.

Besides drilling the flash cards, you can practice sentences in other ways. You can sing songs and read books that contain repetitive sentences. Here are a few suggestions:

Songs
- *Row, Row, Row Your Boat*
- *The Farmer in the Dell*
- *The Mulberry Bush*

Books
- *Clap Your Hands* by Lorinda Bryan Cauley
- *Jump, Frog, Jump* by Robert Kalan
- *Goodnight Moon* by Margaret Wise Brown
- *The Napping House* by Audrey Wood

Thank you for your support. Please call if you have questions or concerns. You are always welcome to observe your child in therapy.

Sincerely,

_____
Speech-Language Pathologist

_____
Phone

Home Practice Log

Child: _____   Speech-Language Pathologist: _____

Parent/Caregiver: Please practice the ABC Flash Cards at the Sentences level with your child daily (at least 5 days per week). Mark a **+** in the box when your child pronounces the sentence correctly; mark a **–** in the box when your child incorrectly pronounces the sentence. Record the total number of correct responses in the box at the bottom of the column. Please return this log when completed or at the end of this phase. Thanks!

Date														
A														
B														
C														
D														
E														
F														
G														
H														
I														
J														
K														
L														
M														
N														
O														
P														
Q														
R														
S														
T														
U														
V														
W														
X														
Y														
Z														
SH														
CH														
TH (voiceless)														
TH (voiced)														
Total Correct														

Sentences

Just for Kids: Apraxia

Home Practice Notes

Parent/Caregiver: Please complete a Home Practice Note after each practice session with your child. Record the number of correct responses from the Home Practice Log in the space provided. Ask your child to return the note to speech therapy for a reward. Thanks!

We practiced the ABC Flash Cards at the Sentences level today.

_____ pronounced _____ sentences correctly!
Child   number

_____   _____
Parent/Caregiver Signature   Date

(Please return to Speech-Language Therapy.)   ☐ Send more notes.

We practiced the ABC Flash Cards at the Sentences level today.

_____ pronounced _____ sentences correctly!
Child   number

_____   _____
Parent/Caregiver Signature   Date

(Please return to Speech-Language Therapy.)   ☐ Send more notes.

We practiced the ABC Flash Cards at the Sentences level today.

_____ pronounced _____ sentences correctly!
Child   number

_____   _____
Parent/Caregiver Signature   Date

(Please return to Speech-Language Therapy.)   ☐ Send more notes.

We practiced the ABC Flash Cards at the Sentences level today.

_____ pronounced _____ sentences correctly!
Child   number

_____   _____
Parent/Caregiver Signature   Date

(Please return to Speech-Language Therapy.)   ☐ Send more notes.

We practiced the ABC Flash Cards at the Sentences level today.

_____ pronounced _____ sentences correctly!
Child   number

_____   _____
Parent/Caregiver Signature   Date

(Please return to Speech-Language Therapy.)   ☐ Send more notes.

● We jumped for joy. ● He ran in a race. ●

● She wants a watch.

Sentences

This is to certify that

_____

has successfully completed

Phase Four of the

Apraxia Therapy Program.

_____
Speech-Language Pathologist

_____
Date

● He ran in a race. ● She wants a watch.

● We jumped for joy. ● He ran in a race. ●

● She wants a watch.

Expressions
Phase Five

Rationale

The final phase of the program, *Expressions: Phase Five*, highlights the rate, rhythm, and intonation of speech. Children with apraxia often speak in a monotonous, careful manner. The prosodic characteristics of speech, which carry so much inferential information, are impaired.

In Phase Five, all aspects of the spoken message are practiced in fun, dynamic expressions. The children are required to tune into the sounds, movement transitions, grammar and syntax, and meaning of the message. Meaning is conveyed not only through words, but also through variations of rate, rhythm, and intonation. This phase should be a lot of fun for the children. They should have sufficient phonetic and linguistic skills to be able to focus on the prosodic aspects of the expression. To help the children retain what they have learned, ask them to repeat easily-produced expressions in role-play situations.

Strategies

Use voice therapy techniques to work on rate, rhythm, and intonation. As with the articulatory aspects of speech production, prosodic aspects must be practiced in exercises with conscious control before they become automatic. The following techniques/strategies will be helpful in Phase Five.

- Continue to use the alphabet signs to cue difficult sounds.

- Provide additional practice for difficult grammatical forms.

- Raise your pitch to over-emphasize specific words in the expression.

- Change the stress on words in an utterance to give it different meanings.
  For example:

      I don't know.
      I **don't** know.
      I don't know.

- Tap out a pattern of beats for the expressions.
  For example:

      Oh me, oh my! (short-long, short-long)

- Chant the expression, exaggerating the normal intonation of the utterance.
  For example:

      Happy Birthday! (low-low-high-mid)

Criterion for Completing the Program

In *Expressions: Phase Five*, all aspects of the utterance are addressed. Articulation, grammar, and intonation should be taken into account when assessing the accuracy of responses. A 75-80% proficiency level should be achieved to complete Phase Five. Phase Five ends the program. It is recommended that each child be retested upon completion of the program to determine an appropriate course of action. Some children may be ready for discharge. Others may need to cycle through all or some phases of the program again. A child may need additional therapy targeting a specific phoneme or grammatical form. You may want to continue with this approach, but in more challenging linguistic and social contexts, similar to fluency therapy hierarchies. These decisions should be made on an individual basis for each child.

Instructional Tools

Oral-Motor Mouth Postures

Pictures of lip and tongue placement for the oral-motor exercises in Phase Five are provided on pages 117 – 118. Use the pictures for additional visual support when doing the exercises.

ABC Flash Cards

The flash cards in Phase Five show an expression and a role play. The expression is the target; the role play is the challenging context. (See pages 119 – 126.)

Supplemental Target List

A supplemental list of expressions is provided on pages 127 – 129 of the manual. Use this list for alternative expressions or additional practice.

Family Letter and Home Practice Materials

The Family Letter, page 130, briefly describes Phase Five and suggests ways for the parents/ caregivers to work with their child at home. Attach a copy of the ABC Flash Cards at the Expressions level, pages 119 – 126, the Home Practice Log, page 131, and Home Practice Notes, page 132. Send these materials home with the children after the first session of the phase.

Phase Completion Certificate

Present the certificate, page 133, to the children when they complete Phase Five.

Phase Five Therapy

Materials
- Alphabet Mouth Postures, pages 139 – 147
- laminated set of ABC Flash Cards, pages 119 – 126, for use in therapy
- Oral-Motor Exercises – Mouth Postures, pages 117 – 118
- small, hand-held mirror for each child
- tongue blades
- reinforcement activity, if needed, page 149
- Apraxia Group Response Form, page 151, or Apraxia Individual Response Form, page 153
- one set of ABC Flash Cards for each child, pages 119 – 126, for practice at home
- one Family Letter, Home Practice Log, and Home Practice Notes for each child, pages 130 – 132
- Phase Completion Certificate for each child, page 133
- Supplemental Target List, pages 127 – 129 (optional)

Session Sequence

❶ Gross Motor Warm-Up

Ask the children to perform a gross motor movement such as running in place, clapping, or doing jumping jacks while singing the ABC song. (See page 148 for additional gross motor movement activities.) Sing the song slowly with exaggerated articulation. Repeat the song and movement activity several times.

> "A, B, C, D, E, F, G,
> H, I, J, K, L-M-N-O-P,
> Q, R, S,
> T, U, V,
> W, X, Y and Z.
> Now I know my ABCs.
> Next time won't you sing with me?"

❷ Oral-Motor Exercises

Ask the children to imitate the following lip and tongue exercises five times each. Display the mouth posture pictures on pages 117 – 118, encouraging the children to match the postures as they perform the exercises. Children may benefit from using their mirrors. Use your fingers to indicate the number of repetitions.

Lip Exercises
- Exaggerate your lip movements as you say, "wah-woo-wee-woo."

- Hold a tongue blade flat between your lips. Try to hold onto the tongue blade with your lips as you pull it away from your mouth.

- Curl your lips in, then push your lips out.

Tongue Exercises
- Lick the roof of your mouth. Start at the "spot" (alveolar ridge) and move back as far as you can.

- Press your tongue tip against your finger or a tongue blade. Push hard with both your tongue and your finger or tongue blade.

- Lick your upper teeth as if getting food off your teeth. Then lick your lower teeth.

❸ Alphabet Chant

Recite the alphabet in unison with the children using the Alphabet Chant found on pages 137 – 138. The chant requires the children to form the sign, say the letter name, and produce the associated sound(s). Use hand-over-hand assistance, if necessary, to form the signs. Show the Alphabet Mouth Posture pictures for added visual support in producing the sounds, pages 139 – 147.

Tips
- Encourage the children to watch your mouth for placement cues.

- Form the alphabet sign near your face to keep the children's attention focused on your face.

- Repeat the sound distinctly three times with a short pause between the repetitions. Prolong continuant sounds, repeating each prolongation three times.

- Present the long vowel sound first, then the short vowel sound.

- The letter C makes the /k/ and the /s/ sound. Present both sounds.

- Present both the voiced and voiceless /th/ sounds.

- Develop a definite cadence to your alphabet review to provide prosodic support.

- Refer to a graphic representation of each letter (e.g., point to the letter on an alphabet chart, place a magnetic letter on a board, use an alphabet puzzle, write the letter on a chalkboard).

❹ Drill Expressions

Drill is the most important factor for success in improving the intelligibility of children with apraxia. The children will come to expect drill as part of the program. Don't let them talk you out of it.

Practice the ABC Flash Cards at the Expressions level. Include practice of the challenging context when the target is easily produced. Record the accuracy of each child's response (+/–) on the Apraxia Group Response Form, page 151, or the Apraxia Individual Response Form, page 153. Use the Supplemental Target List on pages 127 – 129 for alternative expressions or for additional practice.

Tips
- Encourage correct articulation of all sounds in the expression.

- Exaggerate your intonation of the expression.

- Establish a rapid pace of stimulus presentation.

- Elicit a high number of responses.

- Require three to five unison responses, followed by an individual response from each child.

- Cue difficult sounds using the alphabet signs.

- Do not dwell on difficult expressions. Provide a model and production cues, then go on.

- Present the role-play after expressions that are easily produced.

- If necessary, use a simple, quick, tangible reinforcer to keep the children on task. (See page 149.)

❺ Words of Increasing Length

Ask the children to repeat the following syllable groups until the whole utterance has been produced, cueing difficult sounds with the alphabet signs. Use hand gestures to establish an echoing routine. After practicing the whole utterance a few times, call on an individual child to use the utterance in response to the role play. Encourage dynamic expression.

- Ee - Eenee - Eenee me - Eenee menee - Eenee menee my - Eenee menee mynee - Eenee menee mynee mo!

  Role Play: Kyle, you caught a tiger by the toe. What game did you play?

- Hick - Hickor - Hickory - Hickory, dick - Hickory, dickor - Hickory, dickory - Hickory, dickory, dock!

  Role Play: Shiloh, in what nursery rhyme did the mouse run up the clock?

- Pea - Peanut - Peanut but - Peanut butter - Peanut butter and - Peanut butter and jell - Peanut butter and jelly!

  Role Play: Dakota, you love a sticky, gooey sandwich. What kind is it?

- Mar - Mary - Mary had - Mary had a - Mary had a lit - Mary had a little - Mary had a little lamb!

  Role Play: Connor, what did Mary have?

- Shave - Shave and - Shave and a - Shave and a hair - Shave and a haircut - Shave and a haircut, two - Shave and a haircut, two bits!

Role Play: Pedro, what words go along with this (tap long-short-short-long-long, short-short)?

6 Song

Sing a familiar song with the children that has a lot of expression. Sing the song slowly with accentuated rhythm. Cue difficult sounds in key words with the alphabet signs. A rhythmic whole body movement, such as swinging or clapping to the beat of the song, will facilitate precise production of the expressions in the song. Song suggestions include:

Pop Goes the Weasel

"All around the cobbler's bench the monkey chased the weasel.
The monkey thought 'twas all in fun.
Pop! Goes the weasel.

"A penny for a spool of thread, a penny for a needle.
And that's the way the money goes.
Pop! Goes the weasel.
CHORUS

"Rufus has the whooping cough, and Sally has the measles.
And that's the way the doctor goes.
Pop! Goes the weasel."
CHORUS

Zip-A-Dee-Doo-Dah

"Zip-a-dee-doo-dah, zip-a-dee-ay,
My, oh my, what a wonderful day!
Plenty of sunshine headin' my way,
Zip-a-dee-doo-dah, zip-a-dee-ay!
Mr. Bluebird on my shoulder,
It's the truth, it's 'actch'll,'
Everything is 'satisfactch'll.'
Zip-a-dee-doo-dah, zip-a-dee-ay!
Wonderful feeling, wonderful day!"

Bibbidi-Bobbidi-Boo

"Salagadoola menchickaboola, Bibbidi-Bobbidi-Boo!
Put them together and what have you got?
Bibbidi-Bobbidi-Boo!

"Salagadoola menchickaboola Bibbidi-Bobbidi-Boo.
It will do magic, believe it or not, Bibbidi-Bobbidi-Boo.

"Salagadoola means menchickabooleroo,
But the thingamabob that does the job is Bibbidi-Bobbidi-Boo.

"Salagadoola menchickaboola Bibbidi-Bobbidi-Boo.
Put them together and what have you got?
Bibbidi-Bobbidi, Bibbidi-Bobbidi, Bibbidi-Bobbidi-Boo."

❼ Closure

Invite the parents/caregivers into the therapy room. Discuss the session and distribute the ABC Flash Cards, pages 119 – 126, Family Letter, page 130, Home Practice Log, page 131, and Home Practice Notes, page 132. Stress the importance of daily practice and remind the parents/caregivers to complete the home practice logs and notes. Suggest that the family sing the song used in therapy and read the books listed on the letter for additional practice and carryover. The songs and books should be presented slowly and with exaggerated rhythm and expression so the children have an opportunity to join in. Once the child is familiar with the song or book, the parent/caregiver should ask him/her to sing the song or "read" the book without help.

On the last day of the phase, present a Phase Completion Certificate to each child, page 133.

Oral Motor Exercises — Mouth Postures

Lip Exercises

Exaggerate your lip movements as you say, "wah-woo-wee-woo."

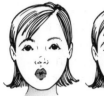 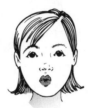 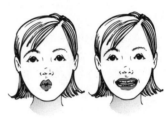 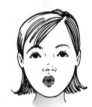

wah	*woo*	*wee*	*woo*

Hold a tongue blade between your lips. Try to hold onto the tongue blade with your lips as you pull it away from your mouth.

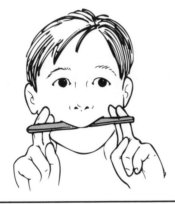

Curl your lips in, then push your lips out.

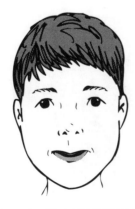 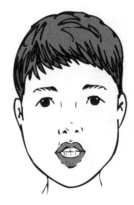

Tongue Exercises

Lick the roof of your mouth. Start at the "spot" (alveolar ridge) and move back as far as you can.

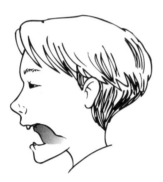 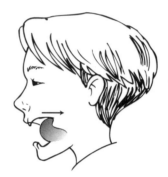

Press your tongue tip against your finger or a tongue blade. Push hard with both your tongue and your finger or tongue blade.

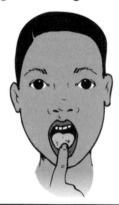

Lick your upper teeth as if getting food off your teeth. Then lick your lower teeth.

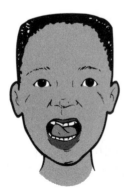 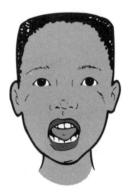

ABC Flash Cards

Now I know my ABCs!

You are proud that you learned
your ABCs. Tell your teacher.

Busy as a bee!

You're getting ready for a camping trip.
Tell me how busy you have been.

Call the cops!

You see a robber in your neighbor's
house. What do you tell your mom?

Hickory, Dickory, Dock

The mouse ran up the clock. Which
nursery rhyme am I talking about?

E

Eeney, meeney, miney, moe!

You have to choose an outfit for the
party. How can you choose?

F

Fee, fi, fo, fum!

You're the giant in *Jack and the Beanstalk*.
You smell the boy. What do you say?

G

Ready, set, go!

You are in charge of starting a race.
What do you say?

H

Happy birthday!

You're invited to a friend's birthday party.
What do you say when he opens the door?

I	J
I don't know.	**Gee whiz!**
You lost your coat. You've looked everywhere. Your stepmom asks you where you put it. What is your answer?	You want to watch TV after school. Your dad tells you to do your homework. What do you say?
K	L
Can I keep him?	**I love you!**
You found a stray kitten in the alley. What do you ask your stepdad?	It's time for bed. You give your mom a kiss and say . . .

M	**N**
Monkey see, monkey do!	**No way, José!**
You and your brother are copycats. What does your grandma say?	Your friend asks to swap lunches. He has sardines. What is your response?
O	**P**
Open mine first!	**Pop goes the weasel!**
You bought a cool gift for your friend's birthday. What do you say at the party?	You turn the handle on the jack-in-the-box and sing the song. Tell me what you sing at the end of the song.

Q	R
I quit! Your cousin likes to beat you at checkers. After losing five times, what do you finally say?	**Ring-around-the-rosey** Your little sister has a favorite game that you play with her all the time. What is it?
S **Sit down, please.** You are called into the principal's office for getting in trouble on the bus. What's the first thing she says?	**T** **Time for bed.** It is 8:00 PM. You've taken your bath and brushed your teeth. What does your dad say?

U

You can do it!

You are up to bat. The bases are loaded.
What do your teammates say to you?

V

Very interesting!

You tell your grandfather about your field trip
to a space museum. What is his comment?

W

We won!

You made the winning home run. The
team is happy. What are they shouting?

X

X marks the spot.

You found a treasure map. How do you
know where the treasure is buried?

Y	Z
Please don't yell.	**I feel like a zombie!**
You yell for your stepmom to answer the phone. What does your stepmom tell you?	You were up until midnight watching a movie. The next day you are very tired. What do you say?

SH	CH
Shark attack!	**Chuga-chuga-choo-choo!**
You're swimming in the ocean and see a shark. What do you yell?	Your baby brother loves trains. What does he say when he plays with his train?

TH (voiceless)	TH (voiced)
I think I can!	**this one or that one?**
The little train is chugging up the hill. It's hard work. What does the train say?	You are in a souvenir shop. You can have one souvenir. Your grandma asks, "Do you want . . ."

Supplemental Target List

Use these expressions as alternatives for the expressions on the ABC Flash Cards or for additional practice.

A — An apple a day keeps the doctor away.
Ask your father.
That's awesome!

B — Bingo!
Put it in the oven for baby and me.
cute as a bug

C — I caught a cold.
Congratulations!
calm as a cucumber

D — a dime a dozen
Don't touch!
You're driving me crazy!
ding-dong

E — Easy does it!
He eats like a pig.
Every cloud has a silver lining.

F — Five, four, three, two, one, blastoff!
Fiddlesticks!
Something smells fishy!

G — fun and games
Go for it!
I'm gonna get you.
Get me out of here!

H — He huffed and he puffed and he blew the house down.
Help me!
Hurry up!

I — It's a small world!
It makes me itch.
That's incredible!

J — Jingle bells, jingle bells, jingle all the way!
Good job!
Jeepers, creepers!

K — Cuckoo-cuckoo-cuckoo. (Say like a cuckoo clock.)
Can I keep him?
kiss and tell

L — Better late than never!
Laughter is good medicine.
Get a life!
Good luck!

M —Money doesn't grow on trees.
Make the most of it.
Maybe yes, maybe no.

N — Never say never!
No more excuses!
nine times out of ten

O — Oh boy!
Okey-dokey!
Open it!
You're out!

P — Pretty pretty pretty please!
Practice makes perfect!
Paper or plastic?

Q — quick as a whistle
as quiet as a mouse
Let's call it quits.

R — Ready or not — here I come!
ring-around-the-rosey
Rain, rain, go away.

S — one step at a time
I feel sick!
Snap, crackle, pop! Rice Krispies®!

T — Timber!
I have a tummy ache.
Tickle, tickle, tickle!
Tell the truth.

U — What's the use?
    Use it wisely.
    Wear your uniform.

V — When she's bad, she's very, very bad!
    Remember to take your vitamin.
    Vvvroom, vvvroom!

W — Watch out!
    Where, oh where, has my little dog gone?
    We'll see.

X — You need some exercise.
    Excellent!
    Too much excitement for one day!

Y — Happy New Year!
    Play in the backyard.
    You are special!

Z — Zip-a-dee-doo-dah.
    It's below zero!
    Slow down! It's a school zone.

SH — Shhh, the baby is sleeping!
    Don't shout!
    Don't shove!

CH — Cheers!
    I like chocolate chip cookies.
    Say cheese!

TH (voiceless) — food for thought
    three blind mice
    I saw the tooth fairy!

TH (voiced) — That's enough!
    The party's over.
    This little piggy went to market.

Dear Family,

Today we began Phase Five of your child's speech therapy program. Your child is learning to produce fun expressions with enthusiasm in his/her voice. Children with apraxia often speak in a monotonous, careful manner. This final phase of our program will help your child commu-nicate the underlying meaning of a message using appropriate rate, rhythm, and stress.

Attached are flash cards with dynamic expressions written on them and some home practice materials. Please practice these expressions with your child. Present the expressions with exaggerated enthusiasm in your voice. Your child will then try to imitate your vocal patterns. If your child begins to mispronounce words, slow your rate, and stress individual sounds. For expressions your child can easily produce, present the role play included on the flash card. It will require your child to retain the vocal patterns of the expression following a short delay. Continue to complete the Home Practice Log and a Home Practice Note every time you drill the ABC Flash Cards with your child.

Besides drilling the flash cards, you can practice expressions in other ways. You can sing songs and read books that contain fun, repetitive phrases. Here are a few suggestions.

Songs
- *Pop Goes the Weasel*
- *Zip-A-Dee-Doo-Dah*
- *Bibbidi-Bobbidi-Boo*

Books
- *We're Going on a Bear Hunt* by Michael Rosin
- *Brown Bear, Brown Bear, What Do You See?* by Bill Martin Jr and Eric Carle
- *Five Little Speckled Frogs* by Virginia Pavelko
- *Five Little Monkeys Jumping on a Bed* by Eileen Christelow
- *Five Little Monkeys Sitting in a Tree* by Eileen Christelow

Thank you for your support. Please call if you have questions or concerns. You are always welcome to observe your child in therapy.

Sincerely,

_____

Speech-Language Pathologist

_____

Phone

Home Practice Log

Child: _____ Speech-Language Pathologist: _____

Parent/Caregiver: Please practice the ABC Flash Cards at the Expressions level with your child daily (at least 5 days per week). Mark a **+** in the box when your child pronounces the expression correctly; mark a **–** in the box when your child incorrectly pronounces the expression. Record the total number of correct responses in the box at the bottom of the column. Please return this log when completed or at the end of this phase. Thanks!

Date														
A														
B														
C														
D														
E														
F														
G														
H														
I														
J														
K														
L														
M														
N														
O														
P														
Q														
R														
S														
T														
U														
V														
W														
X														
Y														
Z														
SH														
CH														
TH (voiceless)														
TH (voiced)														
Total Correct														

Expressions

Just for Kids: Apraxia

131

Home Practice Notes

Parent/Caregiver: Please complete a Home Practice Note after each practice session with your child. Record the number of correct responses from the Home Practice Log in the space provided. Ask your child to return the note to speech therapy for a reward. Thanks!

We practiced the ABC Flash Cards at the Expressions level today.

_____ pronounced _____ expressions correctly!
Child   *number*

_____   _____
Parent/Caregiver Signature   *Date*

(Please return to Speech-Language Therapy.)   ☐ Send more notes.

We practiced the ABC Flash Cards at the Expressions level today.

_____ pronounced _____ expressions correctly!
Child   *number*

_____   _____
Parent/Caregiver Signature   *Date*

(Please return to Speech-Language Therapy.)   ☐ Send more notes.

We practiced the ABC Flash Cards at the Expressions level today.

_____ pronounced _____ expressions correctly!
Child   *number*

_____   _____
Parent/Caregiver Signature   *Date*

(Please return to Speech-Language Therapy.)   ☐ Send more notes.

We practiced the ABC Flash Cards at the Expressions level today.

_____ pronounced _____ expressions correctly!
Child   *number*

_____   _____
Parent/Caregiver Signature   *Date*

(Please return to Speech-Language Therapy.)   ☐ Send more notes.

We practiced the ABC Flash Cards at the Expressions level today.

_____ pronounced _____ expressions correctly!
Child   *number*

_____   _____
Parent/Caregiver Signature   *Date*

(Please return to Speech-Language Therapy.)   ☐ Send more notes.

ZIPPADEEDOODA! • *HIP, HIP, HOORAY!* • I DID IT!

YABBADABBADOOO! • *HIP, HIP, HOORAY!* • I DID IT!

Expressions

This is to certify that

_____

has successfully completed

Phase Five of the

Apraxia Therapy Program.

_____
Date

_____
Speech-Language Pathologist

HIP, HIP, HOORAY! • GIVE ME FIVE! • YABBADABBADOOO!

I DID IT! • *HIP, HIP, HOORAY!* • GIVE ME FIVE!

Phase Completion Certificate
Just for Kids: Apraxia

Copyright © 1999 LinguiSystems, Inc.

Appendix A: Apraxia Assessment

___ **Pretest** (_____)
                       date
___ **Posttest** (_____)
                       date

Child: _____ **Grade:** _____ **Teacher:** _____

Date of Birth: _____ **Age:** _____ **Examiner:** _____

Scoring: +/−

Gross Motor Coordination: Instruct the child to perform the following gross motor movements while simultaneously counting to ten.

_____ clapping

_____ marching

_____ sitting then standing

_____ running in place

_____ jumping jacks

Number Correct: _____/5   **Percentage Correct:** _____%

Oral-Motor Coordination: Instruct the child to imitate the following lip and tongue movements 5 times each.

Lip Movements	*Tongue Movements*
_____ pucker/retract lips	_____ stick tongue out/in
_____ slow kisses/fast kisses	_____ lick top lip/lick bottom lip
_____ hide top lip/hide bottom lip	_____ slow clicks/fast clicks
_____ slow lip pops/fast lip pops	_____ move tongue from corner to corner
_____ press lips together	_____ circle the lips clockwise, then counterclockwise

Number Correct: _____/10   **Percentage Correct:** _____%

Sounds in Isolation: Instruct the child to repeat the letters of the alphabet and the /sh/, /ch/, and /th/ sounds.

___A ___B ___C ___D ___E ___F ___G ___H ___I ___J

___K ___L ___M ___N ___O ___P ___Q ___R ___S ___T

___U ___V ___W ___X ___Y ___Z ___Sh ___Ch

___Th (voiceless) ___Th (voiced)

Number Correct: _____/30   **Percentage Correct:** _____%

C-V-C Words: Instruct the child to repeat the following C-V-C words.

____ bib	____ tight	____ fife	____ shush	____ lull
____ pop	____ dad	____ van	____ chain	____ roar
____ mom	____ kick	____ move	____ watch	____ noon
____ wow	____ gag	____ sis	____ judge	____ hot
		____ zoos	____ thin	____ yolk
			____ them	____ beige

Number Correct: _____/25   **Percentage Correct: _____%**

Multisyllabic Words: Instruct the child to repeat the following multisyllabic words.

____ hot dog

____ dinosaur

____ watermelon

____ hippopotamus

____ kindergarten teacher

Number Correct: ____/5   **Percentage Correct: _____%**

Sentences: Instruct the child to repeat the following sentences. A correct response requires accurate articulation and grammar.

____ I want my hat.

____ He did his homework.

____ She did not do her homework.

____ They like their house.

____ The girl is reading.

____ The boys are playing.

____ The dog hides a bone.

____ The man mowed the grass.

____ The lady found a key.

____ The teacher's helper will do it.

Number Correct: _____/10   **Percentage Correct: _____%**

Expressions: Instruct the child to repeat the following expressions. A correct response requires accurate articulation, grammar, and prosody.

_____ Cool!

_____ We won!

_____ I don't know!

_____ Where are you going?

_____ I want to go home!

Number Correct: _____/5   **Percentage Correct:** _____%

Words of Increasing Length: Instruct the child to repeat the following word groups.

_____ bum - bumble - bumblebee   _____ base - baseball - baseball play - baseball player

_____ fun - funny - funny bone   _____ pea - peanut - peanut but - peanut butter

_____ can - candy - candy cane   _____ birth - birthday - birthday par - birthday party

_____ sub - subtract - subtraction   _____ cook - cookie - cookie cut - cookie cutter

_____ ice - ice cream - ice-cream cone   _____ tee - teeter - teeter tot - teeter totter

Number Correct: _____/10   **Percentage Correct:** _____%

Summary

	Number Correct	Percentage Correct
Gross Motor Coordination	_____/5	_____%
Oral-Motor Coordination	_____/10	_____%
Sounds in Isolation	_____/30	_____%
C-V-C Words	_____/25	_____%
Multisyllabic Words	_____/5	_____%
Sentences	_____/10	_____%
Expressions	_____/5	_____%
Words of Increasing Length	_____/10	_____%
TOTAL	_____/100	_____%

Appendix B: Alphabet Chant

A   The letter *A* says "ā-ā-ā" or "ă-ă-ă."

B   The letter *B* says "b-b-b."

C   The letter *C* says "k-k-k" or "sss-sss-sss."

D   The letter *D* says "d-d-d."

E   The letter *E* says "ē-ē-ē" or "ĕ-ĕ-ĕ."

F   The letter *F* says "fff-fff-fff."

G   The letter *G* says "g-g-g."

H   The letter *H* says "h-h-h."

I   The letter *I* says "ī-ī-ī" or "ĭ-ĭ-ĭ."

J   The letter *J* says "j-j-j."

K   The letter *K* says "k-k-k."

L   The letter *L* says "l-l-l."

M   The letter *M* says "mmm-mmm-mmm."

N   The letter *N* says "nnn-nnn-nnn."

O   The letter *O* says "ō-ō-ō" or "ŏ-ŏ-ŏ."

 P   The letter *P* says "p-p-p."

 Q   The letter *Q* says "kw-kw-kw."

 R   The letter *R* says "r-r-r."

 S   The letter *S* says "sss-sss-sss."

 T   The letter *T* says "t-t-t."

 U   The letter *U* says "ū-ū-ū" or "ŭ-ŭ-ŭ."

 V   The letter *V* says "vvv-vvv-vvv."

 W   The letter *W* says "w-w-w."

 X   The letter *X* says "ks-ks-ks."

 Y   The letter *Y* says "y-y-y."

 Z   The letter *Z* says "zzz-zzz-zzz."

 SH   The letters *SH* say "shhh-shhh-shhh."

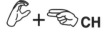 **CH**   The letters *CH* say "ch-ch-ch."

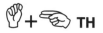 **TH**   The letters *TH* say "th-th-th" (voiceless) or "th-th-th" (voiced).

Appendix C: Alphabet Mouth Postures

Long A (as in *say*)	**Short A** (as in *add*)
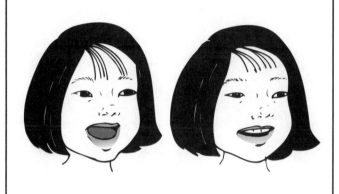	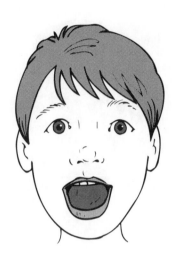

B (as in *ball*)	**C** (as in *cow*)
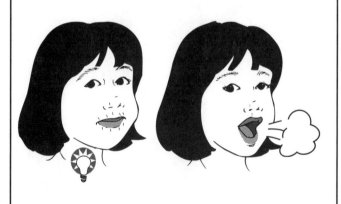	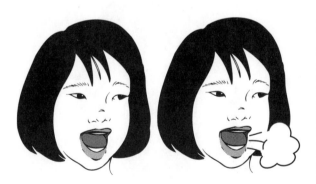

Appendix C: Alphabet Mouth Postures, *continued*

C (as in *city*)	**D** (as in *dog*)
Long E (as in *eat*)	**Short E** (as in *egg*)

F (as in *fish*)	G (as in *gum*)
H (as in *house*)	**Long I** (as in *ice*)

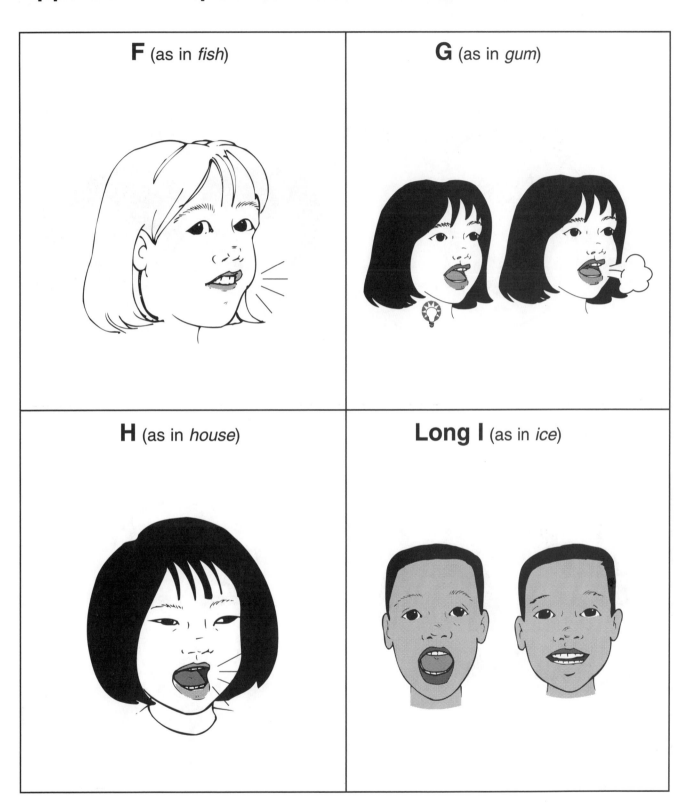

Short I (as in *in*)

J (as in *jump*)

K (as in *king*)

L (as in *lap*)

M (as in *mom*)

N (as in *nine*)

Long O (as in *open*)

Short O (as in *hot*)

Appendix C: Alphabet Mouth Postures, *continued*

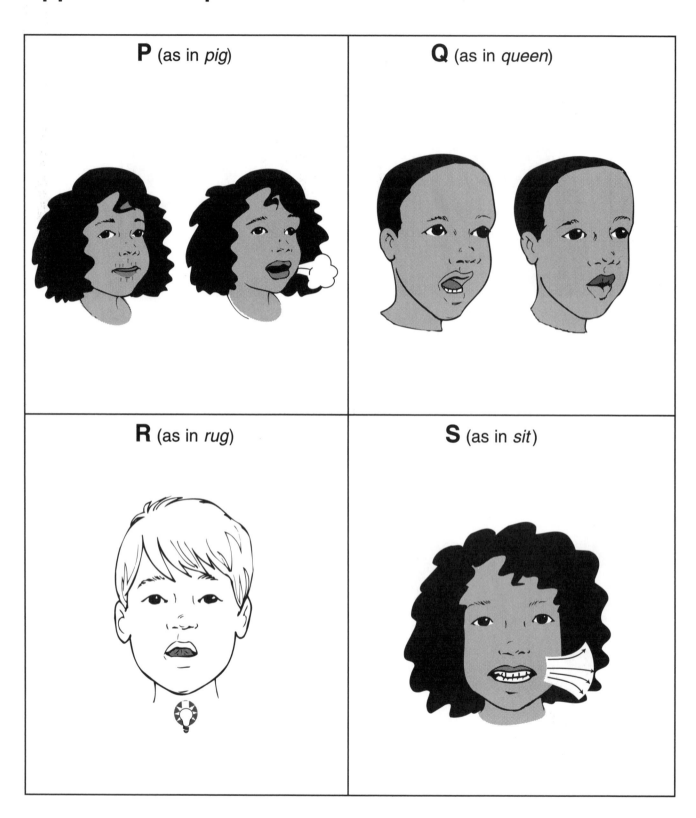

P (as in *pig*)

Q (as in *queen*)

R (as in *rug*)

S (as in *sit*)

T (as in *ten*)	**Long U** (as in *you*)
Short U (as in *up*)	**V** (as in *van*)

Appendix C: Alphabet Mouth Postures, *continued*

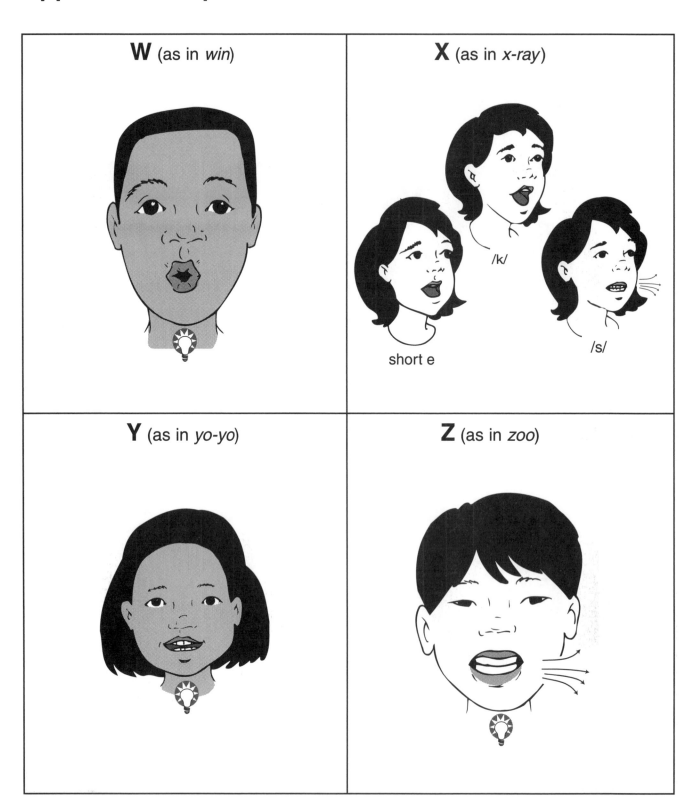

W (as in *win*)

X (as in *x-ray*)

/k/

short e

/s/

Y (as in *yo-yo*)

Z (as in *zoo*)

SH (as in *shoe*)

CH (as in *chain*)

voiceless TH (as in *thumb*)

voiced TH (as in *they*)

Appendix D: Gross Motor Movement Activities

Beginning your apraxia therapy session with a gross motor movement activity will improve the overall coordination of the children. It will prepare them for the fine motor movements required in speech tasks. Listed below are some suggestions.

Low Energy Movements
- clapping
- tapping
- stomping
- marching
- swaying
- hand clapping game
- "Head, shoulders, knees, and toes" song

High Energy Movements
- whole body rolling
- animal walking
- jumping jacks
- hopping
- skipping
- climbing stairs
- spinning
- dancing
- running in place

Movements Using Equipment
- playing hand-held musical instruments
- swinging on a swing
- spinning on a Sit 'n Spin®
- bouncing on a therapy ball
- jumping rope
- punching a bag
- kicking a ball
- balancing on a balance board
- walking on a balance beam
- rolling on or in a barrel
- jumping on a trampoline
- walking on a treadmill
- riding on a teeter-totter
- lifting a parachute
- riding a scooter board

Appendix E: Reinforcers

The most important component of apraxia therapy is drill. The children need a lot of practice to change their motor plans. Most children will do what is expected of them without extrinsic motivators. Some will need a tangible reward to keep them on task. When you find a need for a reinforcer, keep it simple and quick. Save it for the end of the session whenever possible (e.g., toss a puzzle piece into a box for each target drilled, then assemble the puzzle at the end of the session). Below are some suggestions:

- alphabet floor puzzles
- magnetic letters
- foam, cardboard, or wooden alphabet puzzles
- *Window Decorations Alphabet Squares*[1] by Color-Clings
- *ABSeas*[2] by Discovery Toys
- *Mix & Match: The ABC Game*[3] by Smethport
- Duplo® pieces
- blocks
- pieces from a play set (e.g., Fisher-Price Farm, Sesame Street House)
- stickers/sticker book
- stamps/ink pad/stamp book
- tokens to purchase a prize
- peg board
- beads to string

[1] *Window Decorations Color-Clings Alphabet Squares*
Color-Clings, Inc.
P.O. Box 201957
Minneapolis, MN 55420

[2] ABSeas
Discovery Toys, Inc.
Martinez, CA 94553
1-800-426-4777

[3] Mix and Match ABC Game
Smethport Specialty Co.
Smethport, PA 16749

Appendix F: Apraxia Therapy Goals

Long-Term Goal

By _____ , _____ will demonstrate the ability to sequence the sounds and
   (date)   (child's name)

syllables of connected speech while participating in conversations.

Short-Term Goals

- By _____, the child will produce the letters of the alphabet appropriately.
     (date)

- By _____, the child will produce consonant-vowel-consonant words
     (date)
  appropriately.

- By _____, the child will produce multisyllabic words appropriately.
     (date)

- By _____, the child will produce short phrases and sentences appropriately.
     (date)

- By _____, the child will produce common expressions with appropriate rate,
     (date)
  rhythm, and articulation.

Appendix G: Apraxia Group Response Form

Date: _____

Target: _____ Sounds in Isolation   _____ C-V-C Words   _____ Multisyllabic Words   _____ Sentences   _____ Expressions

Scoring: +/–   **Gross Motor Movement Activity:** _____

Reinforcer: _____   **Song:** _____

Name	A	B	C	D	E	F	G	H	I	J	K	L	M	N	O	P	Q	R	S	T	U	V	W	X	Y	Z	SH	CH	TH(vl)	TH(vd)	# Correct/30	% Correct

Comments: _____

_____

_____

_____

Score

# Correct	15	16	17	18	19	20	21	22	23	24	25	26	27	28	29	30
% Correct	50	53	57	60	63	67	70	73	77	80	83	87	90	93	97	100

Just for Kids: Apraxia

151

Apraxia Group Response Form Sample

Date: 10-1-00   **Speech-Language Pathologist:** _Martha Drake_

Target: _X_ Sounds in Isolation   ___ C-V-C Words   ___ Multisyllabic Words   ___ Sentences   ___ Expressions

Scoring: +/−   **Gross Motor Movement Activity:** _jumping on trampoline_

Reinforcer: _alphabet floor puzzle_   **Song:** _Mickey Mouse Club_

Name	A	B	C	D	E	F	G	H	I	J	K	L	M	N	O	P	Q	R	S	T	U	V	W	X	Y	Z	SH	CH	TH(vl)	TH(vd)	# Correct/30	% Correct
Cameron	+	+	+	+	−	+	+	−	+	+	+	+	+	−	−	+	−	−	+	+	+	+	−	+	−	−	+	+	+	+	20/30	67%
Jason	+	+	+	+	+	+	−	+	+	+	+	+	+	+	+	+	+	−	−	+	+	+	+	+	+	+	−	−	−	−	22/30	73%
Kelsie	+	+	+	+	+	−	+	+	+	−	+	+	+	+	+	+	+	+	+	+	+	+	+	+	+	+	+	+	+	+	26/30	87%
Lauren	−	+	+	+	−	+	+	+	−	+	+	+	+	−	+	+	+	+	+	−	+	+	+	+	+	+	+	+	+	+	25/30	83%
Michael	+	+	+	−	+	+	−	−	+	+	−	+	+	+	+	−	−	+	+	+	+	−	−	+	+	−	−	−	−	−	15/30	50%

Comments: _Kelsie — fronting/backing difficulties_

Jason — "biting" description facilitates /f/ and /v/

Score

# Correct	15	16	17	18	19	20	21	22	23	24	25	26	27	28	29	30
% Correct	50	53	57	60	63	67	70	73	77	80	83	87	90	93	97	100

Just for Kids: Apraxia   Copyright © 1999 LinguiSystems, Inc.

Appendix I: Progress Report Form

Child: _____ **Grade:** _____ **Teacher:** _____

Current Phase in Program

_____ Sounds in Isolation _____ C-V-C Words _____ Multisyllabic Words

_____ Sentences _____ Expressions

Student Response

Overall success: _____ excellent _____ good _____ poor

Overall effort: _____ excellent _____ good _____ poor

Rate of success: _____ rapid _____ average _____ slow

Therapy level: _____ nearing completion _____ middle _____ beginning

Strengths:

Weaknesses:

Effective Strategies

_____ watching face _____ matching mouth postures

_____ alphabet signs _____ associating sounds with colored blocks

_____ placement cues _____ clapping/tapping syllables

_____ forward chaining *(b-be-bed)* _____ looking in a mirror

_____ backward chaining *(t-at-cat)* _____ exaggerated stress

_____ slow rate _____ unison productions

Other: _____

Classroom/Home Carryover Activities

_____ recite the alphabet _____ play with alphabet games/puzzles

_____ practice alphabet signs _____ sing the ABC song while _____

_____ practice ABC flash cards *(movement activity)*

_____ sing _____ _____ practice _____ words/flash cards

(song) *(sound)*

_____ read _____

(book)

Other: _____

Comments:

_____ _____

Speech-Language Pathologist *Date*

Appendix J: Program Completion Report Form

Child: _____   **Grade:** _____   **Teacher:** _____

Student Response

Overall success:	_____ excellent	_____ good	_____ poor
Intelligibility:	_____ excellent	_____ good	_____ poor
Self-monitoring:	_____ excellent	_____ good	_____ poor

Strengths:

Weaknesses:

Pre/Posttest Results

Pretest Summary (date: _____)	# Correct	% Correct	Posttest Summary (date: _____)	# Correct	% Correct
Gross Motor Coordination	___	___	Gross Motor Coordination	___	___
Oral-Motor Coordination	___	___	Oral-Motor Coordination	___	___
Sounds in Isolation	___	___	Sounds in Isolation	___	___
C-V-C Words	___	___	C-V-C Words	___	___
Multisyllabic Words	___	___	Multisyllabic Words	___	___
Sentences	___	___	Sentences	___	___
Expressions	___	___	Expressions	___	___
Words of Increasing Length	___	___	Words of Increasing Length	___	___
TOTAL	___	___	TOTAL	___	___

Comments:

Plan

_____ Discharge from Speech-Language Therapy
_____ Repeat the following phases:
    ___ Sounds in Isolation   ___ C-V-C Words   ___ Multisyllabic Words
    ___ Sentences   ___ Expressions
_____ Move to new instructional area:
    ___ Phonology (target phonological processes: _____)
    ___ Articulation (target sounds: _____)
    ___ Voice   ___ Auditory Processing   ___ Fluency
    ___ Expressive Language   ___ Receptive Language   ___ Pragmatics
    ___ Other: _____

Comments:

_____   _____
Speech-Language Pathologist   *Date*

References

Hegde, M. N. *Introduction to Communicative Disorders.* Austin, TX: Pro-Ed, 1991. (Based on N. Chomsky and M. Halle. *The Sound Patterns of English.* New York: Harper & Row, 1968.)

Kusko, C. W. "A Modified Treatment Program for Preschool Children with Developmental Apraxia of Speech." *Journal of the National Student Speech-Language-Hearing Association*, 19-32, 1980.

Prather, et al. "Articulation Development in Children Aged Two to Four Years." *Journal of Speech and Hearing Disorders*, 40, 179-191, 1975.

Rosenbek, et al. "A Treatment for Apraxia of Speech in Adults." *Journal of Speech and Hearing Disorders*, Vol. 38, No. 4, 1973.

Strand, E. A. "Motor Speech Disorders in Children: Differential Diagnosis and Treatment of Developmental Apraxia vs. Phonological Disorders." Workshop on October 7 & 8, 1994 in Lakewood, CO.

Strode, R. and Chamberlain, C. *Easy Does It for Apraxia and Motor Planning.* East Moline, IL: LinguiSystems, 1993.

Strode, R. and Chamberlain, C. *Easy Does It for Apraxia-Preschool.* East Moline, IL: LinguiSystems, 1994.

19-03-9876